Sacred Heart Yoga is a practice that provides an awakened awareness of self to the energy centers on the physical, mental, emotional, and spiritual levels. This practice aids in acceptance of self and the relationship of oneness with Creator. This has given me the opportunity to use specific movements to stimulate energy for greater awareness of divine guidance, greater understanding of my relationship with the Creator, and greater clarity. for manifestation.

— Judy Halliwell

The practice has made me so much stronger. No matter what negative events are going on in my life at the time, I know that everything will work out for the best. I wake up every day feeling so wonderful and grateful that I am alive and so full of joy. I never prayed before; now I pray twice a day and am surrounded with the light of the Christ. I am still challenged by many things in life, but now I know I am not alone.

— Dennis Yesner

I have benefited greatly from working with Virginia Ellen and Sacred Heart Yoga for the past two years. I have been freeing myself from the matrix of my past limited conditioning and have been healing and growing into my authentic, divine self. The practice has empowered me to connect more deeply with my inner divinity, to live it, to surrender to it, and to let go of the outer guru system I had been a part of for many years.

— Suvani Stepanek

I have been a student of Virginia's for over ten years, and doing this yoga practice and healing has transformed my life. I am learning how to love myself, to be kind and gentle to myself. I am experiencing knowing who I really am.

— Andrea Hare

Prior to working with Virginia, I spent years exploring various different healing and spiritual modalities that were clearly important for moving me forward on my chosen path. In retrospect, though, I know now that during those years I viewed myself as completely separate from God and not worthy of unconditional love. Once I began practicing Sacred Heart Yoga, my beliefs and experiences shifted quickly: I now realize that we are all one with the divine and that we can have that unifying experience anytime we wish. Practicing Sacred Heart Yoga brings me a deep inner peace beyond words and an inner knowing that all will be well, no matter what is happening in the 3D world. It's a doorway to purification and unconditional love and the road home to remembering who we really are.

— Shawn Murphy

The Sacred Heart Yoga practice and the course work with [Virginia] have helped me to connect to my divinity and my inner wisdom and strength in ways that continue to enrich my life. My prayer life is forever changed; God is inside of me and always bringing me everything I need moment by moment to take the next step. The yoga has shown me how to access this abundant and life-giving inner resource. I am forever changed and forever grateful.

— Joan Loney

I feel that the Sacred Heart Yoga practice is continually healing and transforming me on physical, emotional, mental, and spiritual levels. Through the Sacred Heart Yoga, I have cleared many deep emotional blocks, healed deep-seated traumatic scars, and experienced powerful insights in my life and an evolution that I believe could not have been attained through any other spiritual modality.

— Mark

THIRD EDITION

SACRED HEART YOGA

Activation of the Sacred Seals

Virginia Ellen with Jesus

Other Works by Virginia Ellen

THIRD EDITION

SACRED HEART YOGA

Activation of the Sacred Seals

Virginia Ellen with Jesus

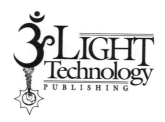

LIGHT Technology
PUBLISHING

For more information about special discounts for bulk purchases, please contact Light Technology Publishing Special Sales at 1-800-450-0985 or publishing@LightTechnology.net.

Sacred Heart Yoga is also available as an e-book from your favorite e-book distributor.

ISBN-13: 978-1-62233-035-5
Published and printed in the United States of America by

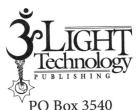

PO Box 3540
Flagstaff, AZ 86003
1-800-450-0985 or 928-526-1345
www.LightTechnology.com

This Book Is Dedicated
to You
and Your Unfoldment

Contents

Acknowledgments xiii

Preface xv

The Second Coming of Christ.. xvi

1   **Steps Along the Path of Working with Jesus** 1

The Value of Inner Guidance 2

The Consequences of Dismissing Inner Guidance 3

Opening to Channel.. 4

Process of Purification 6

Jumping Off the Edge.. 7

A Life-Changing Gift 8

The Christ Within You.. 9

2   **From the Depths of Despair to a State of Ecstasy and Bliss** 13

A Blessing 14

The Hunger for Spirituality 15

A Leap of Faith.. 17

3   **The Transition from Channeling** 21

Ready to Teach 22

The Seven Sacred Seals Hold Your Divinity.............................. 24

Seven Years of Mystery Training with Jesus 26

4   **The Phenomenon of Activating the Seven Sacred Seals** 29
    An Experience of the Activation of the First and
        Second Sacred Seals.. 30
    The Seven Sacred Seals.. 31

5   **The Foundation for the Rest of My Life** 37
    Surrendering to Divine Will... 37
    A Mission in Truth 39

6   **The Yoga of the Sacred Heart** 43
    Sacred Heart Yoga Lineage 44
    A Personal Resurrection into Love 45
    Your Development with Sacred Heart Yoga................................. 46

7   **The Science of the Body**... 47
    The River of Consciousness.. 48
    How Your Thoughts Affect Your Body 48
    Becoming a Christ, God's Ideal of humankind 49
    The Aum 50
    The Aum Exercise... 51
    The Power of the Spoken Word 51
    The Awe of Becoming the Spoken Word..................................... 53

8   **Attunements** 55
    Sacred Heart Yoga Prayer 57

9   **Service to the God Within**... 59
    Service Exercise 59
    Giving and Receiving through Service 60
    Choosing God.. 61
    As I Serve God, I Serve Myself 63
    Meditation in Preparation for Service 65
    How to Use Intentions 65

10 Devotion: the First Stage of Surrender **69**
The Power of Devotion 71
The Divine Flow of Prayers in the First Series of Surrender............73
The First Series of Surrender Postures................................74
Guidelines for Speaking the Prayers 74

11 Purification of the Soul: the Second Stage of Surrender **89**
How the Soul Is Imprinted 90
Release the Need to Control..90
Preparation Exercises..92
The Experience of Awakening the Spiritual Senses 93
Surrender Prayer Exercise 94
The Second Series of Surrender Postures 95

12 The Law of Acceptance **101**
Acceptance Begins the Healing Process 101
The First Phase of Acceptance 102
The Second Phase of Acceptance....................................104
Become What You Want to Manifest or Experience in Life 105

13 The I Am Principle **107**
The I Am Series of Postures 109

14 The Temple.. **113**
The Tabernacle 114
The Tabernacle Posture..115
The Temple of Eternal Life Posture 116
The Temple Flow Postures..117
The First Flow..117
The Second Flow..119
The Third Flow...120
The Mummy Posture..121

15   **The Principle of Desire and Will** **123**

Fulfill Your Desires 125

Desire and Will Exercises 126

The Desire and Will Posture 128

16   **Bring God into Visible Form through**
       Gratitude and Faith **131**

The Path to Attain All of God's Wisdom and Knowledge 132

Faith and Thankfulness 133

Faith Becomes Knowing through Experience 134

Gratitude and Faith Postures 135

Heartfelt Gratitude 136

17   **The Principle of Being** **139**

Being Postures 141

18   **Holy Communion** **143**

The Chakras in Holy Communion 144

Conserve Your Life Force from Leaking 146

The Holy Communion Series of Postures 148

Activate the Fountainhead 151

Enter the Kingdom of Light 152

Epilogue: Experiences Along the Way **153**

Wearing the Garment of Light 155

My Mission in Truth 157

About the Author **159**

Acknowledgments

I am forever grateful to my parents for the gift of life and for giving up so much so that I could have the experiences I needed to learn what was necessary for my own evolution.

I have been so blessed by Jesus and his never-ending love for me, his dedication to my unfoldment, and his daily encouragement. He saw the beauty in me when I was too blind to see who I really was. I thank Jesus for the teachings that I will be sharing with you. They have led me Home, and I now know the divine essence of my being.

My heartfelt thanks to John Kudlak for the valuable gift of his art illustrations. And without the love, support, and dedication of Rosalina Comeau, this book would never have come into form. Thank you for believing in me and in these simple and profound teachings of Jesus. I would also like to thank Cheryl (Ashtara) Concannon for her help in bringing this work to the world. Words cannot express my gratitude to John, Rosalina, and Cheryl for all they have done.

Preface

Jesus gave me so much, and I didn't realize what he was truly giving to me. It took me ten years to put it all together and come to the understanding that I have now. He gave my life back to me to live in freedom and joy. The Bread of Life (light of God) is alive within me now and feeds me each day. I desire in my way, however small or large, to give this gift to you and to have it be available to everyone.

My path with Jesus has led me to many changes within. I now realize that my ego is the part of me that needs to understand the truth of God and the truth of self. My ego needs love and understanding to heal and change its incorrect concepts of self, God, and life. I have learned compassion for myself through the truth that lies within this book. It is a way to evolve into the true Christ-self, the God-self. May you have the pleasure of experiencing your own divine self.

The information that is presented in this book was created to be experienced. Jesus says, "You must experience God to know God. I encourage you to go beyond intellectualizing the wisdom. Go deep into your heart and soul, and feel the words you are reading and speaking."

TEACHING FROM JESUS
It is not what you know about anything that gives you wisdom
but what you know of it that gives it value.

The Second Coming of Christ

The new life and a new world are upon us, and it is the time for the Second Coming of Christ. What is the Second Coming of Christ?

First, it is the time when humanity realizes and experiences their oneness with God. Jesus gave me a direct path, which is the science of prayer and life and living one's life in alignment with universal law. The formula for becoming the living Christ and living in the state of joy and abundance is the gift I am sharing with you.

Second, it is the time for humanity to birth forth the Christ light within by activating the sacred seals. Jesus shares the ancient wisdom that he lived his life by. This wisdom will teach you to become the vibration of God so that the miracle of birthing your own divine Christ light can occur within you.

Third, when the Christ light is alive within you, then you become the conquering Christ. You begin the process of conquering your limited concepts of self, others, and life. Because the Christ light is alive within, you have the ability to transform the energy of your fears into love. This transformation is done at the cellular level, which includes the mental and emotional levels of self. You are being purified by your own divine light. The miracle of your own resurrection from limitation into the unlimited mind of God occurs in the second sacred seal.

Fourth, you will then know who you are, and you will have become one with the noble mind of God. In this state of noble consciousness, you experience equality with others and equality between your own male and female energies. You have gone beyond gender. You are then pure love, pure light, pure wisdom, and pure grace. The I Am will be actively alive within you, expressing your beauty, perfection, and purity.

We are called to ascend and be a living Christ. This is how the Christ will live again within you and me. Our destiny is to become the living Christ. Now is the time, and it is possible for all of us. We are all the chosen ones. We must choose ourselves. If you are ready, make the choice.

CHAPTER 1

Steps Along the Path of Working with Jesus

In 1988, while I was receiving a spiritual energy healing session, Jesus appeared to me. This was my first experience with energy healing. I had never even heard of Reiki or other forms of energy work. Even though I was a complete novice, somewhere within me, I felt this could help me. I desperately needed help. On the outside, I looked as if I had it all together, but on the inside, I was filled with self-doubt and fear.

Zia, an energy healer from Australia, offered to give me a healing. To me, she was extremely evolved, and I trusted her. As Zia worked with me, I entered a deep state of peace and moved into another dimension where all things are possible. She placed one hand on my forehead and the other between my shoulder blades as I lay on the bed. Suddenly, from nowhere, Jesus vividly appeared, illuminated by the light of God pulsating within him and all around him. His crystal clear blue eyes, filled with love and kindness, captivated me. With tender compassion, he spoke: "It is time to lay the cross down."

I was speechless, stunned, and overwhelmed by the power and reality of this experience. It wasn't what he said that affected me down to my very soul. Rather, it was the love that emanated from within him that touched me so deeply. But when I told Zia what had occurred, she acted as though it was nothing extraordinary. As I calmed down, I explained to myself that this must be what happens in an energy healing. When Zia left, I set this experience aside and went on with my life. I had no particular connection with Jesus and did not pray to him. He had no special significance in my life, so I was puzzled.

In the middle of the following week, I tumbled into bed and awoke at 4AM with a burning fever and deathly symptoms that felt like a horrendous flu. By late morning, I couldn't keep fluids in my body. I had nothing in my alimentary tract, yet I could feel each organ beginning to drain as I purged again and again. This continued throughout the day, and by the next morning, I started to feel cold — colder than I had ever felt in my life. Lying there weak, cold, and lifeless, I was dying, and I knew it. I said aloud to myself, "I'm dying."

With this realization, there was relief that the suffering and struggle of my life was finally going to be over. I began to leave my body. There was no fear, just lightness and a sense of peace. Suddenly in brilliant light, there was Jesus. He began talking with me as if he were reviewing my life through a movie we were watching together. I could see myself as a child engulfed by four walls of fear. Jesus told me that during my childhood, I identified completely as a victim with no choice and no chance of getting what I wanted or needed. He explained to me that this perception had created a very low vibration of life energy in me, one loaded with sadness and without hope. Throughout all of the spiritual and emotional work I had done up to this point in my life, I had simply expanded my walls of fear, and I was still living within their confines.

Even though I had spent most of my weekends in self-help workshops and trainings, I apparently had not made any real changes in my consciousness. At this point in my life review, I was shown a box with me in the center. When I thought that I was changing my life, in reality I was just moving from one corner of my box of fear to another. I could never get out of the box and remained confined within the walls of hopelessness and helplessness. I had yet to deal with the real issues — the pain and fear beneath it. I had always accepted what I was given and didn't know I had the right to ask for what I needed. I had evolved as a choiceless person and had yet to address what made me feel choiceless.

Later on during this life review, I remember saying, "Okay, then I can go back," and Jesus replied, "Yes, but you must change every concept that you have lived by."

I was excited by the thought that I could change, and eagerly, I agreed to return. (However, I had no idea what this meant and am still working on changing my concepts of life and self.) Instantly, I felt myself come back to my body and found myself awake and feeling fine. Miraculously, all traces of illness had vanished.

The Value of Inner Guidance

The next morning as I meditated, Jesus appeared again. This time, he took me on a journey into my past and made me face my fears. I discovered that as a little girl, I had decided I was the cause of my parents' endless pain. This decision left me feeling that I had no right to live. Once I could see my belief and feel the pain of it, Jesus told me I had a purpose for being here, God wanted me here, and I had valuable work to do. He said I had chosen this difficult set of childhood experiences so that I would know how it felt to be without emotional support and the nurturing that a child needs to grow. I was a victim to my circumstances. Jesus then said that I was to be a teacher and healer and that my experiences with abuse (emotional, sexual, and physical), divorce, and the death of my three-year-old son were all lessons to help me know and understand the pains of humanity. He taught me ways to heal others and myself along with the spiritual principles that developed into the lessons you'll find in this book.

It was also during this meditation that I learned about the value of listening to guidance. Jesus told me that the first change I needed to make was to sell my bed-and-breakfast business. I worked too hard, Jesus said, and then he gave me practical advice on selling my home business. Since my B & B was located near the site of Ramtha's events in rural Washington, many people were flocking there to hear him. Jesus instructed me to advertise the B & B in a newspaper sent to those attending the events. He set the asking price, which included all that I had originally invested in the home, the remodeling costs, and the furnishings I had purchased to create an adorable country inn. His guidance was that it would sell in six months. Soon thereafter, I had an offer from a lovely woman in Beverly Hills, California, who offered $35,000 less than my asking price. I had a conference with Jesus in meditation, and he said I was not to accept anything less than a fair, full-price offer. I relayed this to my realtor. To my surprise, this woman made a full-price counter offer, but she wanted me to hold a second mortgage of $35,000. Again Jesus advised me to refuse this offer. He said that I was not to hold a second mortgage and that a fair and just full-price offer was coming.

For two months I heard nothing, and I thought to myself, "Well, I blew that one." Then there was a phone call from my realtor with astonishing news. She said that there had been an earthquake in Southern California and that this client from Beverly Hills was offering a full-price cash out for the B & B. It was amazing; I was out of Yelm, Washington, in exactly six months, just as Jesus had said. This was my first experience of listening to guidance and living my life accordingly.

The Consequences of Dismissing Inner Guidance

Now that the house was sold, I needed to find another home for my son, David, and me. The school year had just begun, and David had been elected a class officer. He was also beginning to enjoy success as a star on his baseball team and was planning a trip to Germany with the German club. I decided to give him a choice of returning to California or staying in Washington to finish out the school year. The move to Washington the previous year had been very hard on him, and he had resisted moving away from his California home and friends every step of the way. In spite of his earlier feeling, he chose to stay, and we did.

Jesus had guided me to rent a home instead of buying. All I could find were dark, damp, cold rental homes. Remember, I was from sunny California, and I felt that I was too vulnerable to live in a dark and damp home. There was still so much darkness within me, and I desperately needed light. I didn't listen, and I bought a new home with skylights, light walls, light carpeting, and lots of windows. There was a feeling of warmth and safety in our new home. When tax time came, I abruptly found out why Jesus had guided me to rent a home. The laws at that time did not take into account my first more expensive home in the state of Washington. I had paid much less for my second home there, and I ended up having to pay $30,000 in capital gains taxes on the sale of my California home.

David and I only lived in the home for ten months before returning to California. I had the bright home with skylights for this short time, but it was a costly lesson for me to learn. Since then, I listen to my guidance and usually follow it. When I don't, there is always disharmony.

Opening to Channel

As you can see thus far, each step I've taken on my path (some of which have been very risky) has required a choice that leads into the unknown. Any spiritual path leads essentially into the unknown, and as you travel it, you have to be willing to listen and pay attention to what you feel. In my case, I've found many extended periods of time when there was no clue to the next step. At times, I've felt unready for what's next but have had to do what was asked — that is, make a choice. It takes real desire and strong intention to evolve spiritually. My spiritual path involved taking leaps of faith and had certain costs, some of which may seem not just unreasonable but downright impossible. Jesus assured me that, "Wherever the Father leads you, so shall he be. It is time to begin to rely on the God within, the true source of your good."

Approximately one year after beginning my work with Jesus, I was in my bath meditating with candles and spiritual music. In the meditation, I asked, "Why do I feel so unloved? Why do I feel so separate and lonely?" Suddenly, my body began to flip uncontrollably in the bath water; my hands thrashed, and water splashed all over me and the floor. Jesus merged with me, and he began to answer my questions. He explained why my life had been so difficult. I was meant to heal myself: "Physician, heal thyself!" He then told me that people cannot teach what they have not attained. If you have not learned how to become one with yourself and God, how can you teach others how to become one with themselves and God? Jesus told me that I was to be a teacher and healer. My path was one of self-healing. I was to attain inner peace, understanding, compassion, and love so that I could share this with humanity.

It was during this particular communication that he announced I would channel him in the spring, which was only five months away. My mind screamed, "What, me channel? This is not possible!" I was stunned and instantly fearful, crying out, "Jesus, will my life have to be like yours — full of pain and suffering?" He reassured me that this path did not have to mean a life of suffering.

My mind raced on, thinking how outrageous it would be to channel Jesus. After all, I was a student and a seeker. I was very unworthy. How could I become the one who would channel him? I desperately needed time to think. After mulling it over for a weekend, I decided that if I didn't agree to channel, I would always wonder what I had missed. Besides, I thought that if I didn't like it, I could always stop.

As you can imagine, I couldn't tell a soul. I didn't want anyone to think that I was crazy, so how could I tell people that I was talking to Jesus? It was not long afterward that a friend told me about an upcoming workshop, Opening to Channel. Instantly, I enrolled. I wanted verification that these experiences were true to know that I wasn't making them up or going crazy.

So off I went to the channeling workshop in a picturesque mountain setting near Seattle. There were cabins nestled in the woods and a large meeting room where we gathered. The first evening, all twenty-five participants sat in a circle. The workshop leader was a channel who was clairvoyant, and she went from person to person around the circle describing an entity for each participant to channel. She could see the entities in our energy fields. I had not mentioned a thing about Jesus to her or anyone. As she came to me, my heart flipped and pounded with anticipation. This was the moment of truth. This would be proof that my experiences were true. In that moment, she began to describe a beautiful angel standing behind me, the largest angel she had ever seen. Its presence expanded up to the cathedral ceiling. Immediately, she described another being who came into view and walked toward me; he stood on my right side and wore a burgundy robe. She announced that it was Jesus. I didn't know whether this news relieved me or not. It was just too overwhelming for me to even begin to understand what all this meant.

On the following day, I began merging with the energy of Jesus, bringing him into my body. He always entered on the right. The first time he merged with me, I felt his light move into the right side, and when it entered my heart, this light hit a huge block, causing me intense pain. I felt as if I was having a heart attack, and the pain ran all the way down my left arm. Soon others assisted me by helping move the energy blockage down my arm and out my hand. This healing was necessary so that I could open my heart chakra enough to begin to express the love of this incredible being, Jesus.

On the last day of our workshop, I was resting during the break. Suddenly, I felt as if I had a beard and found myself stroking it with very long fingernails. Muhammad had entered my energy field, manifested in me, and begun to speak to me. He said that I had a large boulder in my heart chakra that he would remove from me that day. I was left reeling from this new experience and all the other incredible things occurring.

As the day wore on, I became numb. I couldn't feel anything. I was so separate from the group, and I didn't feel I belonged. Soon the workshop was over, and the participants expressed their goodbyes with hugs. I went to the man who had shared the workshop flyer about this outrageous weekend with me. He was a large, barrel-chested man. I thanked him, and as he put his arms around me, I instantly started to cry hysterically. In that moment, I felt the large boulder fall to the floor. Muhammad had kept his word. For me, this was my validation that the experiences with Jesus and other entities were real.

Even though I was beginning to accept my experiences with Jesus as real, I was still very uncomfortable telling people that I channeled him. For months after the workshop, I couldn't even say his name. I referred to him as "the entity that I channel."

The Process of Purification

As I continued to practice channeling and merging with Jesus, he expressed that he felt I needed purification. Thus, he put me on a strict diet: no more coffee, sugar, alcohol, soda, white flour, or preservatives. Between merging with his light and the purification of my physical body, I experienced an extraordinary cleansing. My face broke out in bleeding sores that left scars for a time. I then began taking Chinese herbs to support the rebuilding process.

There was other guidance and instruction from Jesus to help me rely on the God within me. I was to leave the material plane and begin to enter the spiritual plane, going beyond time and space into the eternal now. He asked me to put my watch aside, saying that I no longer needed it; then he instructed me to ask myself inside whether I needed to know the time. Jesus also strongly suggested that I disengage from viewing television, listening to music that didn't lift my soul to a higher vibration, and reading newspapers and books. This began the purification from the worldliness I had lived in. As I purified, I began to experience the God within bringing me all the information I needed. If I needed to know something about world events, either the God within me or a friend would tell me. Everything came to me as I needed it.

During my training with Jesus, he also guided me to not work because I needed to spend full days in healing and raising my vibration in order to channel him in the spring. (I learned lessons in trust. I lived on my savings, since there was no money coming in and I still had children at home.) Monday through Friday, my time belonged to Jesus. He would take me on five-day journeys into my darkness, during which I would feel the depths of the sadness and pain within me. On the weekends, I would emerge so that I could spend time with my teenage son.

Jumping Off the Edge

Miraculously, in five months, I made my channeling debut. About thirty curious seekers showed up for my opening night as a channel. Never was I more frightened! My heart pounded so hard that it felt as if it were bouncing out of my body much like a slinky spring, jumping two feet in and out, as Jesus merged with me. During this time of merging, he told me to sound out mystical tones to raise my vibrations and ease the process. He also assured me that I didn't need to know any of the answers to the questions that the audience might have. Somehow, I was able to step aside enough to allow this to occur without difficulty. I don't remember much of what I channeled, but the audience did, and they loved it. They felt his presence. Some even saw his light entering my body, and a few saw his face appear over mine. From that moment on, I had a new career. There was never a need for promotion. People just wanted it.

Within a few months of my first channeling, I was guided to move back to California, this time to the desert area. Jesus explained that the energy in the desert is more conducive to the process of aligning with the Christ-self. I have found the desert to be pristine and to have light where God is visibly present in the naked, natural beauty. Even though the desert was now my home, there were many in the Pacific Northwest and British Columbia who wanted to hear Jesus's wisdom through me. At that time, I was down to my last $1,000 — just enough to pay the rent in the three-bedroom home I had found for my son and my daughter, Michelle, who had returned home to go to college. Jesus had clearly instructed me to continue raising my vibration and to not look for work; instead, I had to trust that the God within would take care of us. Therefore, I spent my days in meditation, in communication with Jesus, and in writing the volumes of his wisdom.

During that time, I traveled to the Pacific Northwest to hold a weekend event. Jesus took me right to the edge, and I jumped off. Just as he had said, God was there to catch me. I then came home with the abundance I needed to provide for my family. Shortly thereafter, one of my Washington participants moved to Hawaii and invited me there. From there, Hawaii participants who later moved to Michigan and Illinois brought me to their healing centers and into their homes. It all just happened effortlessly. There seemed to be a plan beyond my comprehension.

A Life-Changing Gift

Although I worked with Jesus daily and acknowledged his presence for seven years, I didn't express or feel any particular love for him for perhaps the first two years after he appeared to me. In his presence, however, there is no possibility of doubt. Occasionally, I have argued with him and disagreed with what he told me because I found it difficult, but he remains persistent in his messages. Moreover, his messages are always brief and to the point, no explanations added. The messages are phrased or spoken differently, arriving in a language I don't speak. And when they arrive, they touch something deep within.

When I began this amazing journey with Jesus, I had no idea what was in store for me. He would tell me that in the days to come, I would begin to realize the God within and be able to manifest in the moment. This seemed so outrageous, since I was living in relation to the world around me. Something deep within me kept moving me forward, reaching for the miracle of this God that was said to be within me.

Jesus continued to teach me in my seven years of training, and he is still with me even now. I feel that my life and training with Jesus is like being in a modern-day mystery school with initiation after initiation, and this training still continues. He told me that this is the way he was trained, and it is also my path of evolution.

Very often, he gave me specific instruction on how to go about changing my life. The greatest life-changing gift that he gave me was Sacred Heart Yoga. He taught me to use mystical tones to change the physical structure of energy in my body and in the bodies of those around me, and he suggested that I pray and sound out tones as I did each of the specific postures that connected to different chakras. This is how Sacred Heart Yoga was born. I began the process, and as it came into form, I shared it with friends. They too had profound results. This is the Bread of Life, and it allows us to change the incorrect concepts of life, self, money, love, and everything in this third-dimensional world. As we begin to change, the vibrations of our bodies also begin to change. Jesus told me that healing is balancing the energy form of the body. Change the vibration of the body, and the body will heal. Bring forth the correct frequency, and you create the chemicals needed to master your physical body. In so doing, you master your life.

He told me that my physical body was chemically out of balance and that I could use my thoughts to create the correct flow of chemicals for my health. Jesus began to help by correcting me and interrupting me when I thought or spoke in low-vibrational ways. He would stop me and then give me the truth. The first time this happened, I was still living in Washington State. A friend and I had just seen a movie, and we decided to have a bite to eat afterward. I realized that I had been feeling down and lonely because I was single. Suddenly, a low voice interrupted my negative mind chatter, saying, "Be in the moment of now, and be in the state of love. Thank God for your abundance." It felt as if someone had just shaken me. Immediately, I changed my thought flow, which changed my energy to a higher vibration.

I will share a few of his many teachings that helped me tremendously. I hope they will also help you. Jesus gave me his hand, and I now extend my hand to you.

The Christ Within You
JESUS SPEAKS

It is time for the awakening of humankind. I speak to the Christ within you so that you may know your value and your oneness, for I am within all of you. I am the light that shines within all of you. I have come to give you my hand so that you may return home to the beloved Father.

In this oneness and this love lie all things. I shall teach and guide you and take you home to the beauty within you. In your journey home, you shall know the Christ within you. You shall know that which you are and that which you have always been.

It is time to become and express the Christ within you. It is a time of great spiritual unfoldment for all. Heaven is a state of consciousness where you express your divine self through your thoughts, words, and deeds.

Blessed be you who seek the love of God.
Blessed be you, for I love you greatly.

The Magic of God

I speak to you to teach you of the magic of God, to purify your body, mind, emotions, and soul so that you may step forward into the Brotherhood and Sisterhood of God and be a Christ among people. The Second Coming of Christ is within each of you. This is a grand and glorious communion with the light of the Father and the love of the Mother and the divine mind of God. The time has come to move forward, to know your freedom. And so it shall be. Amen.

God's Will

I am with you to teach you the divinity that you are. I desire for you to know that God's will for you is love, abundance, joy, peace, and perfect health, for the Father's will for you is love in all forms, abundance in all forms, and joy in all forms.

Anything unlike this is not God's will for you. The Father's will for you is for you to live in the kingdom of heaven. When you do not allow this flow of love within all of your life, you deny yourself the kingdom of heaven, for then you are entangled in the beliefs and attitudes of the altered mind of ego, the small self.

Anything that is not of love is fear. Any thought or attitude that you hold in fear stops the flow of love in your life. You are then worshipping a false god, the god of limitation and fear.

To begin your journey Home is to begin to notice within you the attitudes and thoughts that you have that are not of love, the thoughts that pass through your mind that are not of joy and thanksgiving. God wills nothing but love for all of humankind. It is your limited thoughts that create a limited life filled with sorrows, illness, and regrets. You can have all things in your kingdom. You are God manifesting in physical form.

Your mind was created to be in Holy Communion with divine thoughts of God, pure thoughts of love and creation. Begin to notice the way in which you relate to life and others.

Do you open your heart and allow the love to flow freely from you? Or are you afraid to express who you truly are? Do you give freely to life and allow life to love and support you? Is your God evil or kind? Does your God punish you?

Whatever you believe is so in your kingdom.
God does not judge you. It is only you who judges you.

When you begin to notice these thoughts of fear, love them and allow them, for they are part of you. Gently give them to the Father. Surrender them into the light. Surrender to the love of God, and allow it to freely flow through you. Do not be frightened of the dark thoughts. Feel the feelings of these thoughts, and then surrender to God's love and light. Allow this divine love to heal you. Do not hide from yourself. Love all parts of you until you are whole.

Blessed be you who seeks the love of God. Peace be with you.

Developing the Christ-Self

As you express the Father within your being, you are developing your radiant body, the oneness with the Father within. As you express in your deed the Father within, you inherit eternal life, eternal youth of this embodiment.

Life is the will of God for everyone.
Death is the will of humankind through its thoughts.

Feed your soul spiritual food of Sacred Heart Yoga, and do not seek the material world, for this shall perish, and you shall be left empty and alone. The Bread of Life (manna) is within you. Let the Father within bring forth the Bread of Life to you, for your spirit feeds you and provides for you.

This Christ-self is God's highest ideal of the perfect man, the perfect woman. It is within all of you. The Christ-self is to be brought forth within each of you.

As you practice your Sacred Heart Yoga and release the power of God through you, you are developing the Christ-self. You come into conscious oneness with God as you serve God. Do not live to please others. In doing so, you destroy yourself. Do not accomplish your goals to prove you are great and brag of your greatness. Achieve your goals for the good of the goal, needing no praise, for you are in service, and all your good comes from the Father within, not the material world or from others outside of you.

To be a Christ, you must be devoted to the Father within, putting this above all other. Be dedicated and devoted to your mission and to expressing the purity of God living through you.

The truth of God is waiting to be lived through you now.

You must be willing
to change your attitudes,
to hold and concentrate on divine thoughts,
to be humble and vulnerable,
to be compassionate with yourself and others,
to trust the Father within totally,
to live for God, and
to allow God to express through you.

When you give yourself completely to God, you live in this world but not of it. You will not be involved in worldly activities, only those that the Father guides you to participate in.

When you give your life in service to the Father within, you have no life separate from the Father. You enter into the kingdom of heaven to share this good with others.

Blessed be you who seek the love of God.
Blessings to the Christ of your being.

CHAPTER 2

From the Depths of Despair
to a State of Ecstasy and Bliss

My first call to change, to expand my consciousness and awareness, was when I was only in my twenties. I was living the so-called American dream: a new home in suburbia and two children, a darling little girl and a precious baby son.

My first son, Warren, was born a few days before Christmas, and I returned home from the hospital on Christmas Eve. When leaving the hospital, he was placed in a large Christmas stocking instead of a blanket. Warren was a Christmas present to all of us from the heavens. This was our own little angel. Joy filled our hearts and souls, and we could truly sing, "Joy to the World." It was a Christmas I will always remember.

A few days after Christmas, I was giving Warren his 2AM feeding. In the silence of the night, my infant son spoke to me with great emotion. I heard his little voice say, "I am going to have a very hard life." Instantly, I began to cry at this message filled with power, energy, and emotion. I felt overwhelmingly scared and sad. Somewhere deep inside of me I knew this was the truth. This was my first conscious awareness of being clairaudient. However, at that time in my life, my mind (ego) couldn't be present with the pain of this message, and because I had not been exposed to spirituality, I had no explanation for this type of communication. I began to rationalize this experience by telling myself that it must be a hormonal imbalance. With that, I stored the experience away to be forgotten. I had no way of understanding what had occurred, and I didn't share this with anyone because it was nowhere in my frame of reference as normal. Also, I didn't want to believe that it could be true; therefore, I went into total denial.

Then, two and one half years later, Warren began to have unusual reactions to light. When I took him out into the sunlight, he began to cry. Soon, he started to wake up sick to his stomach. During these few weeks of signs, I had a dream. In this dream, I was in a hospital, and Warren was dying. I woke up in panic with fear in every cell of my body. Instantly, I remembered the forgotten message. In that moment, I knew that it was all true: My beautiful baby boy was going to be taken from me.

Within a week of my dream, Warren was admitted to the hospital and diagnosed with a brain tumor. At first, I prayed, wept, and pleaded with God not to take him. At that point in my life, I still believed God was outside of me somewhere in heaven with a long beard and a staff.

You read about these things, never believing that they will happen to you. Well, it was happening to me, and I was forced to feel. I felt helpless as I watched my son deteriorate. I wanted to stop the endless hours of what, to me, was torture. I became extremely angry with God and the Catholic Church. There were no answers, no compassion or kindness in the priest with whom I sought counsel. The only answer I received was that this was God's will. Who was this God who would make a child suffer so? I had a million questions about life, God, and religion. I left my church because the God I was raised to believe in was useless to me now.

Warren's illness lasted nine months. There were six surgical procedures and numerous radiation treatments. The pain was overwhelming to me. My heart was torn apart. As I write this, there are tears in my eyes. I am still healing and embracing the truth that Warren hasn't left me and that he is with me always. I have the ability to communicate with him, so I know that this is true. Yet some part of me is still holding on to wanting him here to hold and love in the physical form. I am just now beginning to be willing to let the pain completely dissipate.

A Blessing

After my son Warren's death, my husband and I decided to adopt a child. We investigated the possibilities, and they were very bleak. We went to many different adoption agencies but did not find a suitable match. We gave up on adopting a child.

On the first anniversary of baby Warren's death, God answered my prayers. A college friend of my husband's, who had adopted a baby boy through an attorney the year before, called. A miracle had just occurred: The attorney had just called to tell our friend of a baby boy who had been born that morning at UCLA Medical Center. The attorney asked whether the couple wanted the child. Our friends weren't ready for another baby and told the attorney about us. I immediately thanked them and called my husband at work. The next day we were on our way to Beverly Hills to see the attorney. She took all of our history and said she would be giving the mother five families to choose from. Neither doubt nor hope was in my mind. I just let it go to focus on handling my emotions from the loss of Warren.

Since this was the weekend of the anniversary of our son's death, we planned to go away on a holiday with our daughter, Michelle. We were trying to create a normal life again for our family, so we went to our favorite hideaway, a ranch-style resort called Warner Springs in Southern California. I was soaking in one of the large outdoor mineral pools at the resort when I was paged. Running to the phone, I couldn't imagine who would be paging me. When I answered, I received a message that changed my life forever. The attorney said that the baby was ours and that we could pick him up at the UCLA Medical Center anytime we were ready. Overwhelmed with excitement and joy, I shared the news with my husband and then with Michelle. She began jumping up and down, saying, "I won't have to be all alone anymore." It had been a very hard two years for all of us, especially for Michelle. She had no way of understanding why her life had changed so dramatically.

The next step was to call my brother and his wife to share our blessing. I asked them to buy some diapers and bottles since we were ready to pick up our new baby boy and bring him home with us.

We left early the next day for UCLA to get our son, David. There, I experienced my second cosmic encounter with the mystery of God. David was premature, weighing only four pounds and six ounces. As my husband and I stood in front of the viewing window, I felt and saw a light leaving my heart chakra, and I saw a light leave my new infant son's heart. The two lights met in the center of the hospital nursery, and I said aloud, "That's him!" We instantly bonded in that cosmic moment, and I never once had any fear that the birth mother would change her mind. He was my son, and I knew no one could ever change that. He is a child of my heart and from the light. It took six months to finalize the adoption. David was a blessing to all of us, helping us heal the wound we all had felt so deeply.

The Hunger for Spirituality

The death of my son Warren had created a tremendous amount of change within me. Four years later, I found myself dissolving my marriage. This inspired greater growth. I was faced with the fears of being alone, and for the very first time, I had to take care of myself as well as my two children. I wasn't prepared for this extraordinary challenge. Having married very young, I had gone from my parents' home right into marriage.

The fears that came up were almost unbearable. The fear of being alone was particularly excruciating. My lowest point came one morning after I sent my children off to school. Very suddenly, a movement of agony came up within my body and out of my mouth as I made inhuman noises while clawing my fingernails along the wall. I sought out counseling, which was my saving grace. I had fallen apart to such a degree that if I hadn't had that one-hour weekly session with my counselor, I would have perished. I often thought of suicide. It was only the thought of my children needing me that kept me going on. The counselor was a spiritual woman who suggested that I read certain books. The first one that I read was written by Wayne Dyer, which changed the course of my life. As I read, I saw myself in all of my dysfunctional behaviors. It was then that I made a commitment to myself to become whole. I hungered to know God, to know love, to know happiness, and to know peace. The hunger inside of me was so great that I devoured numerous books with their spiritual teachings.

At that time, I didn't realize that a strong intention and a great desire could create so much change or evolution in life. However, with my strong commitment, I began to evolve.

I attended the Erhard Seminars Training (est) at the urging of my counselor. She said participating in the training would help me release my sense of victimization. I had no idea what est entailed, but I followed her guidance and enrolled. This training led to the transformation of my relationship with my father. In one of the processes, I suddenly saw, for the first time, that my father was in desperate need of my love and kindness. The next time I saw him, I reached out to him and was able to put my arms around him and love him unconditionally. This was the first time I ever felt this kind of love for him. In that instant, something happened, and he felt my love. Our relationship changed, and we became best friends.

The next step in my evolution was to become involved with the local Church of Religious Science. There, I learned to meditate, and twice a week, I attended yoga classes to begin to heal my back. Soon I became a workshop junkie, trying everything that came along. I tried rebirthing, breath work, hypnotherapy, Rolfing, and exercises from the Science of Mind I and II classes. Each of these modalities helped me move forward to release my walls of fear and limitation. My spiritual path consumed me and brought me the first real peace I had ever known.

During these years, I developed a fashion consulting business and was very successful. The classes and training were paying off. My life as a single woman was fulfilling. I was finally finding myself. I wasn't just a daughter, a mother, or a wife. I was creating my own life and loving it. Life was good, and I prospered.

It was during this time that I read Shirley MacLaine's book, *Dancing in the Light*, a fascinating work. Shirley introduced me to channeling and the entity called Ramtha. I distinctly remember saying aloud, "I have to know about this" and then feeling a rush of energy throughout my body in every single cell. Within a week, I took a friend to church, and we visited the bookstore after the service. There, on the shelf, was a single book entitled, *Ramtha: The White Book*. Instantly, I took the book off the shelf, thrilled with my discovery. My friend saw my excitement and bought the book for me. God was truly working in my life and leading me to the next step.

I couldn't wait to begin the adventure of discovering this new information. Reading this material was profound for me. I was unfamiliar with the language Ramtha used, but more importantly, the message was beyond my understanding. I had to read some of the pages two or three times to get the meaning. But at a deep level within me, I knew the information was the truth. I recall saying, "This is why I came to life." I also knew deep within me that this would be my path. I read the book four times in six months, and each time, I felt that I had never read it before. Each time, my understanding of the truths contained within the book grew.

I stopped going to my church. Instead, I spent my Sundays alone in my backyard gardening and communing with God. I began to hear messages of truth that brought me greater understanding. I knew I had found something precious, and I treasured these moments of oneness with God.

A Leap of Faith

After these Sunday experiences, I decided that I needed to find out more about the Ramtha teachings. I called Ramtha Dialogues in Washington State and found that they would be having a four-day workshop in the California desert in December. It would be just around the time of my birthday: the perfect gift. I enrolled, and off I went, leaving the children with my mother for the five days. I said to her, "I don't know where I am going, but I will never be the same."

The most significant experience of the week for me was when I went out into the desert, climbed up on a rock, and went inside myself in meditation. I can't recall what I said once up on the rock, but suddenly my heart chakra opened. It felt like someone had cut my chest open with a knife. What came out was sadness, and I just sobbed and sobbed. When I finally stopped, my chest closed, and I felt lighter. I climbed down my little mountain and journeyed back to the retreat center.

Something happened up on that rock, and I came back different. I continued to seek Ramtha messages through video and audiotapes, and visited the center in Yelm, Washington, for a private audience with the master. It was during this trip that I decided to move to Washington and follow my spiritual path. This was an enormous decision for me. I had lived in my California home for twenty years. I had never been separated from my family and friends. Something inside of me, a force that I can't explain even to this day moved me. I sold my home in two weeks and walked away from my prospering business. My daughter, who was nineteen at the time, refused to join me, so I had to leave her behind, but I took my son with me. My family and friends cried and then became angry with me. There was no support from anyone. Yet this force inside of me kept urging me forward.

The day I left California and began my drive to Yelm, Washington, was the first time I felt fear about this change. As I drove, I began to cry. Fear of the unknown had overcome me. My mind was going crazy with doubt, remorse, and regret.

When we arrived in Yelm, we moved into our new home on fifteen acres of land. I had never lived in the country before or in a cold climate. David was angry with me and resisted finding any good in our new life. I knew no one, I had no job, and it was very cold. It snowed the first morning after our arrival and I had to walk out to a shed to gather wood for the wood-burning stove so that we could have heat. I cried all the way back to the house — the fashion queen was now carrying wood. I was used to being well coiffured and dressed in designer clothing. My life was certainly different now.

One day, the fear overwhelmed me. After David left for school, I curled up in the fetal position in my bedroom and cried, not knowing what to do or where to turn. This experience in Yelm was the second hardest time of my life, yet the most rewarding. The death of my first son had created massive change, and now being alone in this rural area and having to face my fears lead to my transformation. I have found that my hardest times in life have also created the most good. In the moments of those hardships, I could never have imagined where the experiences would take me. I believe now that our hardships bring us closer to God and closer to ourselves. I see them as being in divine order.

I continued to evolve, and this was the time in my life when I was guided (in meditation) to start my bed-and-breakfast for those coming to hear and see Ramtha teach. There were no hotels in Yelm, just a few diners. There was no flash, no beauty, and no fun. But my bed-and-breakfast was an instant success. Visitors from all over the United States and even from overseas came to stay with me to be a part of the Ramtha work and teachings.

I planted a garden for the first time in my life and enjoyed watching the magic of food growing from seeds. I was such a novice at all of this. The fresh experience of opening leaves and finding that cauliflower growing in the center was amazing to me. I was like a child in wonder of nature.

I now realize that in order for me to be reached by Jesus, I had to move out of the structure of my so-called perfect life. I was always on the go and busy, busy, busy. My days were scheduled six months in advance. When I arrived in Yelm, I felt as if someone had dropped me in the middle of nowhere, in a land without schedules. Now I realize that I used to be like a hamster going around and around on a wheel, unable to stop. Divine Spirit certainly put a stop to that way of life. There now was plenty of time to be with myself and in nature.

My encounter with Jesus taught me how to become all the things Ramtha talked about. He started me at square one and took me step by step into higher and higher states of consciousness and bliss. He gave me a simple way to master myself and taught me to master my mind, my emotions, and my body. He gave me the truth, the way that I had been seeking. The intention and desire I had spoken in my bedroom when I first began my journey was manifesting for me.

I now know the ecstasy of God's love for me. Yes, God brings me to such highs that I literally have orgasmic experiences. The state of bliss is normal, and the pleasure of God moving through my body is an everyday occurrence. This is available to everyone. It is our natural state. I continue to evolve into the truth. I still continue to heal my limited self through this path of evolution. There is no destination. It is a forever awakening to more love, to more joy, to more self-respect, to more self-love, and to more pleasure.

CHAPTER 3

The Transition
from Channeling

In 1994, the days of channeling were coming to completion for me. Jesus explained that in order to develop as my own Christ-self, I needed to rely only on the Father within me. I had begun surrendering my own personal needs and desires through devotion to God as Jesus had suggested. In the first series of Sacred Heart Yoga, postures and prayers are utilized to bring a sense of oneness with the Divine. The Sacred Heart Yoga system is a transformational experience of your beliefs or concepts, your emotions, your soul, and your cellular structure. Each of the eleven phases has a specific purpose. During the time I was transforming, I was focusing on the initial phase. As I continued to work with these techniques of movement, sound, intentions, and prayers, something extraordinary began to happen. At first, I felt energy moving throughout my body as a great sense of oneness overcame me, creating a sense of peace I had not known before.

After a few years of sharing this method with others, however, something even more profound occurred. One day, as I walked through the grounds of Rosario Resort on Orcas Island in the Pacific Northwest, I noticed the abundance of wildlife. Deer and fawn even came up to me to eat out of my hand. It was a warm summer day, a perfect outside setting to an inner experience into unknown realms of spirit. I was there in the Northwest to lead a spiritual retreat because Jesus had requested I teach in an environment that lent itself to the participants becoming easily absorbed without distraction in the energy for a period of time. I taught yoga in the morning and channeled in the afternoon.

On the fifth day, when I sat down to begin the yoga postures and prayers with my retreat participants, something different happened. Suddenly, while I was in the

Holy Communion sitting posture, I spontaneously began a singing chant. I don't sing! It was as if it wasn't me. Something overtook me and began to express spiritual wisdom using me as a vehicle. I was in the experience when my ego popped in and said, "What the hell are you doing?" I realized that I had just revealed the most sacred part of myself to others. It was a horrifying feeling. I became overwhelmingly embarrassed. It was as if I were standing naked in front of an entire group. I opened my eyes to see whether anyone noticed. Peeking through, I saw that the entire group appeared enraptured in their own experience of bliss. I was so relieved. But in my head, I asked Jesus, "What is going on?" and he replied, "The Father was speaking through you as you." I had become my spirit.

This experience of allowing Spirit to express through me has continued. It is truly a state of bliss. In these moments, I feel complete with no needs or wants.

A year passed. Sitting on my patio in the desert of Southern California, sunbathing in "my office," my favorite place, I had an overwhelming sense of how wonderful my life had become. I was comfortable and quite content. And then I heard his voice. Jesus said, "It is time to move to the Big Island of Hawaii and expand. Take nothing with you." I thought Hawaii and expanding sounded really good. I moved.

I had heard that Hawaii can cleasne you, especially the Big Island where legends of Pele, the fire goddess, become reality. I found them to be real. Pele is the great goddess of transformation, and so it was for me. The change from the Southern California environment of country club living and malls contrasted sharply with the remoteness and simplicity of island living. There were few shops and fewer distractions. In the beginning, I found myself homesick and wanted to know when I could leave. I was told I needed to stay a year. It was an adjustment for me. When I settled in, however, I found that I could sit on the beach for hours and just be. The pace was slow, and I found myself not as motivated as usual. I could see the differences in energy and consciousness from an environment obsessed with business, money, personal appearance, and hectic schedules as compared to a life of just living. I grew to discover the joy of letting go, especially of my personal image.

Ready to Teach

Shortly after settling into life on the Big Island of Hawaii, I found myself leading another retreat at Kalani Honua Conference Center in the rain forest. It was May, and the air was warm and balmy. Walking across the grounds to the hale (Hawaiian for "house"), Jesus spoke to me, informing me that I would not channel at this retreat. "What am I supposed to do with all these people for seven days?" I asked. He replied, "Lie down, and everything will come from within you. You are ready to teach." This was no comfort to me. Instead, it felt more like a bomb had just been dropped on me.

I took a deep breath and walked into the hale where twenty-six participants from all over the United States and Canada had gathered to hear Jesus's profound wisdom. While the group sat on their yoga mats and waited, I stood up and announced what had just occurred while walking across the lawn. Fortunately, they were all very supportive, though they wondered what would happen next. I too wondered this.

Feeling as if I had no choice, I obeyed and lay down. I was so stunned from what had just happened that I couldn't even begin to imagine what was about to occur. There wasn't time to think, so I began the postures and prayers of Sacred Heart Yoga. To my amazement, the energy began to move my body so profoundly that my legs bounced rapidly up and down in what I later learned is called a "kriya." A kriya is an involuntary response or movement. As the light (energy) moves through the body, it hits blockages in the energy channels that cause the body to jerk or twitch. My abdominal muscles also began to contract as if in childbirth. It felt as if I were being consumed by the light of God. With this movement, a breath began to breathe me. The energy moved up my spine through my chakras (vortexes of energy located in the subtle body) and out the top of my head. With this, I went into a state of ecstasy. It was as if the divine energy was making love to me within, caressing and bringing me to higher and higher states of ecstasy. This energy felt very sensual and orgasmic in nature. This phenomenon went on for the full seven days with the experiences gradually intensifying and building over the week.

During this incredible week, infinite wisdom seemed to effortlessly come forth from some previously unknown part of me. I had never heard this information before. The knowledge of sacred seals and activating the brain just came forth as it was occurring for me and the group. Jesus has told me that this experience is the birthing of the Christ light within. It has since happened for many while practicing Sacred Heart Yoga and during Sacred Heart Therapy sessions.

It was a totally outrageous week. During many of the yoga sessions, states of ecstasy apparently overtook various members of the group. It may have sounded as though we were having an orgy. This energy pouring en masse through the group created orgasmic sensations for everyone. In the next hale, another workshop was in session. They heard the sounds of ecstasy coming from where we were, and at lunch, they jokingly invited themselves to join our group, saying they wanted whatever we had. None believed that our sounds were in response to praying.

I myself felt in awe of what was happening. I had never dreamed I could experience so much pleasure and bliss in the physical by praying, much less be in an entire room filled with people experiencing the same thing. I have realized since this retreat that the human body is created to experience pleasure and not pain. This is the value of relying on the Father/Mother presence within me.

The Sacred Seals Hold Your Divinity
JESUS SPEAKS

You are not truly living until you activate the life of God within. You will then live in alignment with God's laws. Through the process of activating the sacred seals within, I have found the kingdom of heaven, my divinity in each chakra. The sacred seals are located above the chakras. They are chambers of energy lying dormant, waiting to be birthed into life.

Within each sacred seal is an aspect of your divinity, and each has a divine purpose. Once you activate the divinity that is sealed within the chakras, one by one, it is as if you have a new computer. This computer is within you, and it is operated by your thoughts, prayers, sounds, and feelings, which bring forth your grace, beauty, power, knowledge, love, and more — all from within. Essentially, it is all that you need in any given moment. God is alive within you, waiting to be experienced and expressed in this dimension.

As this new foundation is developed and solidified, you hold a new vibration within you. Currents and waves of energy are released from the first seal, sending out a new energy flow that affects the entire system. These waves of electrical energy are sent up the central nervous system to activate the brain, which can bring about full enlightenment. These new currents and waves of energy also develop and expand the DNA system. Once the sacred seals begin the activation process, you create a new foundation for your life, the foundation of a Christ or a fully realized being. The energy of the Divine Mother within you (your Shakti) begins to heal you. The Mother knows exactly what is next on your path to enlightenment; you just need to ask. She transforms the distorted energy to return you to balance, love, and light.

How to Activate the Wisdom of the Sacred Seals

Beloved of God, stand in the pureness of your tears, your sadness, and your anger and fears, for through this shall come the pureness of your love. The gateway to your spiritual body is through your emotional body, beloved ones. You and only you can open the doorways that are barred shut within. Behind these doorways lies your great sadness. This sadness is your passageway to your spiritual body, to your supreme love, to the supreme God that lies within you waiting to be birthed.

You have been crying out for assistance. You cry out for your God powers. These powers are needed now on your plane to restore balance and harmony, first to you and then through you to the world. There are many who are ready to activate the power of God that lies dormant within them. There are those whose intentions are pure and whose services to God and humanity are great. These beloved ones shall not abuse this power. Now is the time for you to be given the power of the God that lies dormant within you.

My beloved ones, within your sacred seals lies dormant a great energy. It is your power. The glory of God resides within your sacred seals. As each seal is activated, the God/Goddess within the seal becomes a live embodiment within you. Once all seven of your sacred seals are fully activated and releasing their specific energies, you will have the power to manifest exactly what you desire in your kingdom in the moment. Each seal releases a current of energy unique unto itself, on your demand, to bring forth manifestation. This energy of God is lying dormant within each seal, waiting to come to life and live through you.

It is as on a cloudy day there is darkness. It is dreary. It is dismal. You know that the power of the Sun exists; however, it is not felt or seen in the moment. You are lost in the fog, lost in the storm, yet in your awareness, you remember the life qualities of the Sun. You do not have the power to command the Sun to bring forth its life-giving radiance.

There is within each seal the power of the Sun waiting to come to life, to clear your body, emotions, and mind of the storm of anger and clear the dark clouds of sadness. Once the activation begins, the power of the golden Sun within the sacred seals begins to clear the atmosphere and your body, mind, and emotions. As you clear the storm within, the power of God — the golden Sun in each seal — becomes stronger and stronger until it is pulsating life through you.

One fine day, beloved ones, you will stand strong and tall. You will put forth your intent, and so it shall be. Each sacred seal will bring forth the precise energies needed for manifestation. You will indeed be powerful and aligned to God's will for you.

I bring you the gift of activating your sacred seals. Look within; feel and know whether you are indeed aligned to the evolution of life. Are you aligned in service? Is your intent pure? If you are indeed aligned and your service is pure, then come forth for the activation of your sacred seals. It is time that the God power be present on your plane. There is need in the density of your dimension for the power that is within you to be activated.

It is within you. You have been told this for eons, and now you are being given the gift of activating that which is within. And so it is. Amen.

Seven Years of Mystery Training with Jesus

When I agreed to be a channel for this work that Jesus asked to deliver through me to humanity, he requested seven years of my life. He said that it would take seven years of purification for me to begin to hold the Christ vibration. I accepted this mission, which he calls, "a mission in truth," bringing the truth of God to humanity.

Those seven years were like living in a monastery — very different from the life I had known before but normal for a mystery school. There were no books, no television, no newspapers, no normal relationships with males, and no outside interference from the world. Everything would have to come from the God within me. I had to rely on God and become as God is. I was challenged and tested over and over again as I continued to dissolve the ego. With time, I began to more feel deeply not only my deepest sorrow but also the joy of my own essence. (Today, I feel as if my body is a highly fine-tuned instrument and that it is being played constantly, as I feel the light moving throughout my entire being. Whenever anything is said or done to me or to someone in my presence, I feel the pleasure or pain of the intent behind the words or actions.)

Throughout these years, I lived very isolated from society, and I was consumed with the project of the transformation of my body, mind, and emotions. I didn't have a community to interact with. I didn't join in or participate with others in classes because I was traveling two weekends per month doing channelings and classes. When I was home, I was preparing for the next trip and healing myself, which was my major project. I had to attain the new information and cellularly embrace it before I could teach the next phase of mastery. There was no time to create a life in the community where I lived.

The finale to these seven years was a retreat in Hawaii over New Year's Eve. The name I was given for the retreat was "The Feast of the Passover," which Jesus says means passing from the material plane into the spiritual plane.

Each day that I led the Sacred Heart Yoga, my vibration would continue to increase. I became very ill with a high fever and head congestion, and I had difficulty eliminating the fluids from my body. Jesus said these symptoms would last ten days because I had begun to embody the Christ vibration, and major purification was occurring. And in ten days, I was completely healed of all discomfort and symptoms of illness. The amazing part about these highly transformational experiences was that when I was teaching, I would have no symptoms of illness. My body was sustained by the light within me. As soon as I finished teaching a session, I again became overwhelmingly ill and returned to bed until the next session. This miracle occurred over and over during the retreat.

I finally finished my seven-year commitment to Jesus. Now I could have my life back. I went on strike. No more teaching. I was free to attend a local church, take yoga classes, enjoy church retreats, and develop friends in the community. I loved my new freedoms, especially when it came to being a student and having no responsibilities. I had a life, but I didn't know what I wanted to do, and my money was running out.

CHAPTER 4

The Phenomenon of Activating the Seven Sacred Seals

When you activate your sacred seals, you will be purified in body, mind, soul, and emotions. The Divine Mother energy within will cleanse you of your pains, guilt, shame, and karma. You will begin to purify, and your healing, directed by the Mother, will take its own course. Your healing will be cellular, very deep and very profound.

As your sacred seals activate and grow in strength, your body will go through many changes. You will truly have a physical and energetic phenomenon occur within your physical body. The light of God is electrical, and it will electrify your physical body. During this electrifying experience of your sacred seals activating, you may experience the following:

- Your head may be moved back by a force of energy from within you. It may feel as if it is pinned back and immovable. This is the state of surrender in which you physically give your body to the God within.
- Your chest may also be arched and held up by the energy for a period of time. Remember, you have surrendered to the force within and are not in control here.
- For both men and women, the muscles in your second chakra area will begin to spontaneously contract as in a birthing experience. This is the Divine Mother energy birthing the light within.
- A spontaneous breath will begin to breathe through you, moving the energy up the main channel through the chakras and sacred seals, exiting the top of your head, clearing blockages, and saturating each cell with love and light. While you

move through these blockages, you may experience states of pleasure (heaven) and pain (hell). In one moment, you may feel the ecstasy and bliss of the light of God tingling and caressing every cell of your body, and in the next moment, you may hit a blockage and feel the pain of an experience stored in the soul record of your body. You may even have a flashback, viewing the experience as it is dissolved by the light.

This phenomenon of awakening and activating your sacred seals, or the Divine Mother energy, may last about thirty minutes during which the body is continually moving in and out of states of pleasure and pain. Spontaneous surrender postures and breathing will continue throughout this time. The pleasure of the Divine Mother energy may heighten, and you may find yourself making sounds of ecstasy as in lovemaking. The senses are being awakened and purified as the body is being cleared of past experiences.

Upon completion of this birthing process, every cell in your body will be alive with God's life. You will feel more sensual than ever before. A sensual being is one who is alive, awake, and illuminated with light — sensitive to life, self, and God.

This is a very natural, mystical experience with your own divine nature. All of this divine mystery occurs as a result of our devotion to God, our willingness to surrender to God and into our own darkness, and our great willingness to trust God throughout this whole process.

An Experience of the Activation of the First and Second Sacred Seals

In September of 1997, a student of mine came for a Sacred Heart therapy session, during which the Divine Mother within me said that this was the day we would activate the first of her sacred seals. I was given the prayers to bring forth her divine Christ light into life. What follows is her description of the experience:

Activating my sacred seals was a divine experience, and my words will not do it justice. With a full and grateful heart, I will attempt to convey it.

Prior to this experience, I had been practicing Sacred Heart Yoga for about a month. Each practice was unique in that more and different energy would vibrate through my body, bringing with it a new awakening each time.

When I say "vibrate through my body," I mean a movement that my conscious mind had not initiated — perhaps the shaking of an arm or leg that leads to the abdomen and up the spine and out of my body. This is a divine feeling and always leads me into peace.

This particular day, I did my yoga practice and then went to receive a healing session from Virginia. When I got on the healing table, Virginia shared that this was to be the day for activating my first and second seals. I was excited, thrilled, and honored, and there was the doubt that it might not happen. All this was swirling around in my mind as the session began. At first, I could only feel the incredible warmth and love energy coming through Virginia. Then I remember being shown my own internal and external light (that flame of energy held deeply within us all that always is). My breathing became spontaneous as if in labor. Many times my body moved and shook rapidly. The light became so bright at this point that it held me in a 360-degree egg, and it showered through every cell in my body.

After this, there was a time of bliss I had not known before. As the breathing and movement continued, it became more intense, calling forth a powerful energy within my womb — but what? This, for me, was the experience of birthing and being the Divine Mother. At this point, I asked for the help of Jesus Christ, and immediately he was in front of me. He put his arms around me and held me. He showed me that he lives within me, that he lives within us all. We are all actually what is meant by the Second Coming of Christ. It is within us, held in our bodies and our hearts.

My own birth of the Christ light occurred in 1993 in a retreat setting. Today, the birthing and activation of the Christ light is available to all those who are ready to receive it.

The Seven Sacred Seals

I would like to share with you the divinity of the chakra system. The chakras are more than vortexes of energy. The sacred seals are the crowns of the chakras. Within each sacred seal lies the divine male and the divine female aspects of God. This is where the power of God lies, where the transformational energy for healing lies, where the wisdom and knowledge of God lies. This energy lies dormant within each one of us, waiting to be activated. There is a divine purpose and function for each sacred seal. The divinity within each sacred seal is the vehicle to activate the brain for full enlightenment and to expand the DNA system. It is the power and glory of the Christ, the kingdom of God within.

The First Sacred Seal

Location: base of the spine
Color: red
Divinity: female aspect — the Mother of Creation
function — the flow of inspiration and divine ideas

male aspect — the passion to manifest
function — the passion to manifest and fully live your creation; to put inspiration and divine ideas into action

The first seal is the life force center. When this sacred seal is activated, you will find the eternal flame within it. After activation, the color becomes a fiery red and begins to burn away the old, limited consciousness within the cells, and energy moves up through your central nervous system into the brain to activate and awaken it.

The Second Sacred Seal

Location: midway between the pubis and the navel
Color: orange
Divinity: female aspect — the Divine Mother
function — to transform energy

male aspect — the beloved Father
function — to protect, to provide for, to bring wisdom and guidance

This seal is the transformational center, and when it is activated, you will have the power to transform your energy, thoughts, emotions, and physical body. As you come home to the Mother and bring your feelings and issues to her, she transforms them through love. The womb of humankind is found in both men and women. Transformation occurs within this womb. New energy is sent up through the pathways to every cell in your body, transforming them from density into light.

The Third Sacred Seal

Location: between the navel and the base of the sternum

Color: yellow

Divinity: female aspect — the desire of the Goddess

function — to desire and ignite the flame of God's will

male aspect — the will of God

function — to bring the desire into form

The third seal is the generating center. The Goddess in you does the desiring. If the desire burns within you, then the Goddess within ignites the will of God, and God generates the Goddess's desire into form quickly. The function of the male is to serve the female. One of the ways he serves her is through honoring her desire and bringing it into form quickly.

The Fourth Sacred Seal

Location: center of the chest (heart center)

Colors: green (healing), pink (self-love), gold (divine love)

Divinity: female aspect — the queen

function — to reign in her queendom in a state of joy, expecting good

male aspect — the king

function — creating a safe, supportive, joyful, and abundant life so that the queen can reign in joy

The sacred heart is the seal of living in the queen- and kingdom. When you are the queen in your kingdom, you enjoy life without lack, worry, doubt, sadness, and needs. You can expect all of your needs and desires to be met effortlessly. Life is lived in the moment of now, and the past is complete. This is joy, the paradise of emotions. When the lower seals are each in balance, you live in joy. In the first seal, the male creates his domain through passion to live the female's creation. He does what he needs to do to put it into form. In the second seal, while the womb transforms the emotions and issues, he provides protection and cares for the physical needs of the feminine. He gives the guidance you need to move forward in your emotions and issues. In the third seal, he honors your feelings, desires, wishes, and needs. Having done all of this, he has provided the domain in which the female can reign in joy.

The Fifth Sacred Seal

Location: at the throat

Color: blue

Divinity: female aspect — the priestess
function — fearless determination

male aspect — the priest
function — speaking the truth

This seal is the state of deliverance, a state in which all things are possible and delivered to your doorstep. Everything already is in the fifth seal. It is exciting because your first four chakras are in balance, and your creative idea is now delivered to you. Your feminine aspect has already had the creative thought. You have transformed the fear or doubt about it, and you have desired and emotionally felt it. In your heart, you are living the joy of the idea. Now, because you are living the joy of the idea, it will be delivered to you. Your male aspect has done whatever he needed to do. He has provided the passion to manifest the feminine creation and protected, cared for, and guided you through the transformational time. In the third seal, he honored your desires, and in the fourth seal, he created a domain for you. Therefore, he could speak the truth about any of the former, saying whatever is necessary

The Sixth Sacred Seal

Location: middle of the forehead

Color: all colors and all hues (the blending of all that you are and the evolution of your soul coming into physical form)

Divinity: female aspect — the maiden
function — to be pure in body, mind, and soul

male aspect — the knight
function — to live in honor

In this seal, honor returns to you. The knight lives by a code of honor. He knows what correct action is and lives accordingly. The knight is the lawgiver in his kingdom and lives according to his laws, honoring the maiden and protecting her purity. As the knight in you develops, you become the conqueror of your kingdom. When the sixth sacred seal is activated, you begin to live as a true mystic. At this level of spiritual evolution, there is no longer a veil, allowing you to see clearly. You must have been extremely healed; otherwise you would not be able to stand the pain of what you see in the souls of humanity.

The Seventh Sacred Seal

Location: crown of the head

Color: purple and lavender hues representing royalty, white light representing divinity as a human God

Divinity: female aspect — the empress
function — to know the truth and govern her empire in love and joy

male aspect — the emperor
function — to know the truth and govern his empire in love and joy

This seal is also known as the knowingness center. You are a noble being. To be noble means to know that you are God, to know who you are, and to live in the truth without limitations. You have resurrected your consciousness and live in the noble mind of God. In this state of noble consciousness, you experience oneness and equality between the male and female aspects of God within. There is no gender in this state of being. You are pure love and light, pure God and human. You know you are entitled to live in the abundance of God's kingdom. The empress and emperor have joined in one truth; they have one focus, they hold one intention, and they unite in one commitment and one desire. They merge into oneness, and at this point of union, there is no gender. They have become pure divine intelligence, pure divine truth and love, living in bliss. This truly is the ultimate in the tantric experience.

CHAPTER 5

The Foundation for the Rest of My Life

One day while in yoga class, a voice (my inner child) said, "Let's go to yoga camp." Immediately after class I went to buy a yoga journal, and I found that there were dozens of yoga schools offering certification programs. So I decided to get certified while learning more about other forms of yoga. I chose a school that two of my Sacred Heart Yoga students had attended. The time was right, and I just needed the money to make it happen.

Jesus said that this time at yoga camp would be the foundation for the rest of my life. This intrigued me, but he never explains these comments, leaving me to find out through experience what he's talking about. He also told me that I would have the money, approximately $3,000, for the month-long yoga training.

The time was growing close, around the time I called my uncle to wish him a happy birthday. To my surprise, he said, "I hear you want to go to school."

"Yes," I replied, "but I don't have the funds yet."

"It's in the mail," was his answer. Thanking him for his support, I began to cry. "That's what uncles are for," he replied.

Surrendering to Divine Will

I put all my belongings into storage, and off I went into this adventure. I found the work interesting, since I had never been exposed to a guru or any Indian philosophy. I enjoyed learning about their traditions and their religion. Chanting was enjoyable, as was learning more about the asanas, or postures. Classes were held seven days a week from 7AM until 5PM, with later evening sessions as well. I was used to being disciplined, so the demanding schedule didn't bother me. However, after two weeks of Sanskrit, I was hitting a wall of resistance. I longed for the sweetness of prayer and toning with my Sacred Heart Yoga and the bliss it brings me.

That morning during the yoga class, I kept hearing, "Do not put false gods before you." So I began sounding with my asanas and saying my prayers from the heart. Later in the morning, I worked with a partner doing the matsyasana, the fish asana, and when it was time for her to assist me during my turn, I told her, "I have to do this my way." I then said my prayer of surrender, and my body spontaneously began to move up into the fish, then back down, and I began to bounce several inches off the ground as the energy of the prayer moved through me. This had happened before, but my partner had never seen or felt anything like this. The instructors were amazed at the Shakti, or Holy Spirit, moving through me.

After lunch there was always a period of chanting; this day we did the Hare Krishna mantra. I decided to chant "Christ" instead. Fifteen minutes into the session, I allowed the Holy Spirit to take full sway of my body. As it took over, moving through me, I felt great pleasure. Suddenly, from deep inside my gut (the third seal) my voice said, "Lord Jesus, you are my Lord and my God, and I will only follow you." Tears streamed down my face. My body began to vibrate at a frequency so high that it took me into full orgasm, releasing sounds of ecstasy. The energy moved from my first seal up through my body, my chakra system and seals, and out the crown of my head, whipping my body back and forth as if I were a rag doll. Upon completion of the movement, I fell exhausted to the floor. Then I realized what had happened. Seventy students and our instructors were looking at me shocked and wondering what that was all about. I pulled myself up from the floor, embarrassed yet so filled with bliss that it really didn't matter whether they understood the mysteries of God moving through the human form.

Even though I had worked with Jesus as my teacher and guide, I had never surrendered to him. A part of me, my ego, always held back, wanting to be in control and wanting life my way rather than God's divine will for me. When I proclaimed him as my Lord and my God, I surrendered my life and my allegiance to him and pledged to follow my divine path to completion. I had finally surrendered to fulfilling my mission.

After that moment, Jesus manifested and spoke to me for the remaining two weeks of my training. He told me that I would write a book and share Sacred Heart Yoga with the world. This yoga was a vehicle to birth forth the light of God, the Christ light, within humanity, and it was part of the movement of the Second Coming of Christ. Sacred Heart Yoga was a way to ignite that light. He also told me that when enough of us held the vibration of the Christ, he would come again. Jesus went on to say that we are the Second Coming and that Christ resides in all of us.

I completed the month-long training for the certification program, and it was time for my final test: leading a yoga class to other students as a teacher observed and graded me. The night before my final, my stomach was in knots, and I couldn't sleep. During a personal healing, I discovered that my stomach was in knots because I was nervous about losing my integrity. I felt that it was impossible for me to lead the yoga as I had been trained for the past four weeks, so I decided to teach from my truth, what I knew within me was the truth. I also decided that I was willing to fail my final test and leave without the certificate. Keeping my self-respect and my knowing was what was right for me. To me, no compromise was acceptable.

As I taught my fellow students in practice sessions, my body would go into spontaneous kriya as the Holy Spirit moved through me. The instructors found this unusual, and they were probably frightened by the movements. One or two of them would try to stop me from my experience by placing their hands on my shoulder or knee and asking me to be still. For the final test, I was the last one in my group to lead. When my turn came, I led the yoga from within me, speaking wisdom about each posture. This was not part of the program that I was training in. When I had completed leading the students, my grading instructor said to me, "A good teacher knows her material. A great teacher knows her material and teaches from within herself, and you are a great teacher." To my amazement, I passed. My grading instructor asked me how long I had been teaching. I told her, and shared that I also had a videotape of my Sacred Heart Yoga, which she later purchased. God had sent me the perfect grading instructor, one who resonated with the energy I represented.

A Mission in Truth

Next was my mission in truth. I was guided to go to Hawaii and teach. While there, I stayed with Rosalina, who was the first person I had certified to teach Sacred Heart Yoga. As we walked on Kailua Beach (our favorite), I shared my mission with her, and she agreed to assist me. The water was many shades of blue that day. As we walked and talked, I remember saying, "Well, I have no money and no resources to begin writing a book and starting a school. It's going to be interesting to see how this all unfolds." I saw this project as a great adventure into God's plan for me.

I returned to California to visit with family. One day while doing my Sacred Heart Yoga meditation, I asked Jesus where I should live. He replied that I should return to the California desert. Then I asked him how to do this, since I only had $100 to my name. Again, I received an answer: "You will stay with Mary." Mary was a young woman I had met at a church retreat just before leaving the desert. We had an instant connection, and I had also performed a healing on Mary after the retreat. During this healing, Jesus merged with us and became a large part of Mary's healing and life.

As soon as I received the message from Jesus about staying with Mary, I called her. Her words to me were, "I redecorated the guest room. The key is waiting for you, and you can stay as long as you like." I was blessed again with God's love providing a home to live in and a sister on the same path with me, a path into God's kingdom.

I began to establish myself by doing healings at a spiritual resort and health center and teaching yoga classes. I also returned to my church. One evening after a church meditation, I shared my mission of writing a yoga book with the group. An artist friend, John, who was there volunteered to do the artwork as a gift to me. We began the project, and he also told me that there was an apartment available in the complex he managed. At that time, I wasn't financially prepared to move. However, I looked at the apartment, and it was quite adorable. But I had to tell him the time wasn't right and thanked him for considering me.

One month later, Mary decided to move to the Los Angeles area, and I went off to lead a yoga certification program in Hawaii. During a yoga session, God told me to call John and inquire about the adorable apartment. It had been six weeks since he had shown me the apartment, and the likelihood it was still available was low. It was winter in the desert, the most desirable time to be there. When I called, the apartment was still available. I returned home, and as Mary made her move, so did I. However, I was faced with the challenge of having to triple my income to meet my expenses.

After moving into the apartment, I was guided to give notice at work so that I could do all my work out of my home. I was petrified as I gave my notice. That evening I did some Sacred Heart Yoga and prayed. I asked God to take the fear out of my body so that I could follow my path. God took it away. Each day of that first month was an adventure into God's abundant life. The phone would ring, and I would be asked to do a massage or a healing. Somehow, I created enough to meet my new expenses.

Two years later, in January 1999, I was leading an evening workshop called New Beginnings. The class was on manifestation: to live a new year cocreating our lives as we choose. Near the end of the workshop, I lead the group into proclaiming their truths and desires. This was a process of accepting the truth from the soul. From within me came a prayer and declaration: "I am ready to take my work into the mainstream." I had never consciously thought or said this before.

Five days later, I received an astonishing phone call from a friend I had not seen in nearly five years. Cheryl said she was heading to the desert for some rest and asked whether I was available to have lunch with her. The following week at lunch we visited, and I also arranged to have a dinner party for Cheryl and several other friends who knew me from my earlier channeling days.

Cheryl had attended my channeling debut with Jesus eleven years previously. We were old friends, and she was also the person who invited me to channel Jesus in Hawaii, where she had a home. After dinner, we were all chatting, and Cheryl said, "I want to help you with your book. My husband is the founder of one of the largest literary agencies in the country." At the time, I didn't even know there were literary agents. However, I soon had an agent, and my book would become a reality. I began the project of getting my book ready to publish.

It was spring, and Jesus once again guided me to give up my home to go be among the people. I put everything into storage at the end of April with no plans for the summer or fall. To my awe, God sent me many invitations to speak and teach all across the nation, from California to South Carolina.

When I began to bring forth Sacred Heart Yoga as a form of devotion, I did not know where it would lead me. However, I did know that my life was with God, and I had no life separate from God. At this moment, I feel an overwhelming sense of gratitude for the love that I have found and for the joy of resurrection through this mystical path of yoga. I bless you and join you in your personal resurrection into love.

6

The Yoga of the Sacred Heart

The mystical form of yoga and prayer that Jesus shared with me has blessed me. This ancient practice of the sacred heart was part of mystery school training. While participating in the yoga of the sacred heart, you will develop your spiritual gifts and activate your sacred seals. Within the heart chamber (one of your sacred seals), you will find many gifts of the Holy Spirit. The greatest gift I have found is my sacred heart, where the true union with God is. Your connection to higher intelligence is also found in the sacred heart. As you live within your sacred heart, your DNA will expand and your physical body will regenerate. There is always unconditional love, mercy, compassion, forgiveness, and understanding in your sacred heart, which is the heart of God, the heart of the Christ. The Christ-self is lived through the heart. The sacred chamber of the heart is the magnetizing center of our lives. It is our use of love that brings to us our good, which we sometimes call good karma.

As I have diligently immersed myself in this beautiful form of mystical prayer and yoga that I originally named Shakti yoga, I have been developing my sacred heart. The sacred heart is the holy of holies within me that I heal from, pray from, and manifest from. And this holy place is within all of us. As the sacred heart is activated and developed, we become the living Christ. This is the Second Coming of Christ. It is the love of God actively living and expressing through each one of us.

I would like to share a holy experience with you. In December 2001, I taught a healing class to several of my Sacred Heart Yoga teachers. One afternoon at lunch break, I was resting and praying when suddenly my third eye opened and I entered eternity. I saw a brilliant blue sky with the most beautiful white clouds I had ever seen. Suddenly, a path was made for me, and I felt my whole body moving through the void, just like a near-death experience I had in 1989, except that this time there was light everywhere. I continued my journey, and at the end of the path, there was a crystal light. When I entered the crystal light, Jesus said I was in the sacred heart and that the ancient practice he gave me had led me there. He shared the wisdom of the sacred heart with me and told me that I could now lead others into the sacred heart within them.

The next moment, my students were knocking at the door. They entered the room, and I remained lying on my bed while I shared my experience with them. I took all of them into the sacred heart to begin healing from this place of love. They all easily entered this holy sanctuary within themselves, and I continued to share the healing practice with them.

This sacred moment in time was so precious. Before then, I wasn't sure how to teach the method of going within the sacred heart. God provided the way. Since that day, I have renamed the yoga and my healing work. It is now called by its rightful name: Sacred Heart Yoga and Sacred Heart Healing and Therapy. I encourage you to begin this ancient practice so that you too can enter, activate, develop, and live within your own sacred heart. The world needs your higher intelligence and unconditional love now.

Sacred Heart Yoga Lineage

Sacred Heart Yoga is given to us by Jesus from the lineage of the House of David and the House of Abraham. Jesus says that "house" means consciousness and that this yoga is from the highest order of the I Am consciousness. For generations, the men and women from the House of David and the House of Abraham used simple devotional prayer in their yoga practice to attain God-realization, much like those used today in Sacred Heart Yoga.

Students on the yogic path pay homage to their lineage and are connected to the lineage through their teachers. Students (devotees) are devoted both to the path (the teachings) and to the teacher (guru). The key to connecting to the lineage is heartfelt love and gratitude. Following is an active meditation for connecting to the lineage.

Become still and focus on your heart seal, feeling the love within. Then begin to let your love flow, gratefully feeling your love and devotion to her. Next, feel your heartfelt love and connection with Jesus and with Joseph, Jesus's father and teacher. Continue to acknowledge and feel your gratitude for all the men and women of the House of David who followed this way. King David was from the House of Abraham. Now begin to feel your love and gratitude for all the generations of men and women from Abraham's House who attained I Am consciousness. Ask the lineage to feed you in your practice and on your daily path of attaining higher consciousness. They know the way and are available to guide you, love you, and nurture you.

A Personal Resurrection into Love

Sacred Heart Yoga is a personal resurrection into love. Jesus says, "Resurrection is to live fully without limitation." This practice engages all of you. It captures your mind, heart, body, and energy. Each time you practice Sacred Heart Yoga, you dive deeper into the soul, into the self. It is a multilayered process. Each layer of your limitation moves into freedom, and then that layer is resurrected into love.

Sacred Heart Yoga is a practice that unlocks the wisdom of the body while activating the brain and the sacred seals. Your soul, mind, body, and emotions experience purification. Sacred Heart Yoga accelerates your spiritual awakening. This practice allows you to bypass the intellect and enter your sacred heart, where you will experience eternal peace, higher intelligence, blissful love, and oneness with your divine essence. Jesus was a master of yoga. He lived and demonstrated the true essence of yoga. Sacred Heart Yoga includes all the forms of yoga listed below:

- **Bhakti,** a yoga of devotion and love. It purifies the emotions and brings peace to the soul.
- **Gnana,** a yoga of knowledge. It educates the intellect and brings forth self-realization.
- **Hatha,** a yoga of asanas, or movements. It serves the body and generates relaxation, flexibility, and strength.
- **Karma,** a yoga of service. It helps you live in alignment to the highest and best for you and your contribution to life. It heals the pains of the past.
- **Kundalini,** a yoga of the spine and nerves. It stimulates the energy system and brings forth enlightenment.
- **Laya,** a yoga of mantras, or prayers. It thrills the nervous system and raises and quickens vibrations.
- **Pranayama,** a yoga of breath, which moves energy through the body. It clears the body and emotions.
- **Raja,** a yoga of meditation. It creates stillness and peace.

- **Sahaja,** a yoga of surrender. It provides purification and opens the gateway to ascension.
- **Tantra,** a yoga of relationship with all aspects of self. It weaves together the divine male and divine female within, the intellect and emotions, and the body and spirit. Union and wholeness is experienced with all aspects of self, and the kundalini is awakened.

Your Development with Sacred Heart Yoga

As you practice Sacred Heart Yoga, you will develop your ability to focus and be in the moment, fully experiencing what is within. You will learn to feel whatever emotion and whatever truth is there in the moment — be it love, joy, peace, sadness, or pain. With consistent practice, you will learn that you can move easily from the darkness into the light by being real and humble and by expressing your feelings to the Indwelling God. You will no longer resist the darkness but will choose to surrender into the darkness.

You will begin to trust the divine Source within you to bring forth the perfect prayers for you. The next step will be to choose to trust God to bring you whatever you need in other areas of your life. If God can answer your prayers, God can bring you anything you need in life. The ego mind of doubt and judgment will begin to dissolve as you trust this source to speak the words of truth and love. The God of your being will then begin to speak through you, as you.

Remember to be in the moment, and above all, be real when speaking the prayers. Use my prayers only as a guide. Your development is based on speaking your own prayers of truth. Each time you lie down to begin your Sacred Heart Yoga (which speaks directly from your heart to God within you), your prayers will have their own life and pattern. Unfold naturally by speaking what is in your heart and soul in the moment.

CHAPTER 7

The Science of the Body

Sacred Heart Yoga is based on the science of the body as Jesus brought it to me. Begin to think of everything as vibration rather than as good and bad or right and wrong. We are drawn to people, places, and things through vibration. We attract to us people and experiences by the vibrations we send out to the world.

Thought is electrical and vibrates at its own frequency. Vibrations are the language of God. In other dimensions, communication occurs through sound, color, and symbols. They all hold consciousness and vibrate the frequency of consciousness through the sound, the color, or the symbol. We communicate consciousness through the spoken word and through art, writing, music, dance, and movement here in this dimension.

Your body lives within its own atmosphere of thought, which is your electrical field, or aura. Beyond your aura, which is filled with color, is a pure energy of white light that is your spirit. Your spirit is one with the mind of God. The mind of God knows all there is to know. Superconsciousness is one-mindedness — the Infinite Mind of God.

Your spirit brings you electrical impulses from the mind of God. What you think determines which impulses will come to you. You draw to you vibrations that match your thoughts or frequencies. In Sacred Heart Yoga, you tap into the Infinite Mind, which brings high frequencies that purify the atmosphere around you, your body, and your soul. The atmosphere around your body is made up of vibrations from both your conscious and unconscious thoughts. This atmosphere is a reflection of your attitudes about life, about yourself, and about others.

Your body holds the past in it. It holds the vibrations of the material plane, which are your human appetites for pleasure. Jesus says, "If you choose to pleasure your body (your animal soul), you will know all of the pains of hell." This statement refers to all of our human appetites for instant pleasure, such as drugs, cigarettes, alcohol, food, money, and sex. It is when we are addicted that we know the pains of hell. We have the opportunity to dissolve the addictions and their vibrations in Sacred Heart Yoga.

The River of Consciousness

There is a river of consciousness that feeds you. It is the river of life force energy that flows through the central nervous system to support life in every cell of your body. Your consciousness creates and conducts the flow of this life-force energy.

You send back to the mind of God the frequencies of the thoughts that you have embraced through your soul. When you live in service to God, your soul releases power and love, which are of higher frequencies. If you choose to serve the mind of the body, the material plane, you send back to the mind of God a lower frequency.

Each thought that you hold has a different frequency and vibrates at its own rate; the purer the thought, the higher the frequency. Jesus says, "When you are pure in thought, you are one with God."

Everything that you think and feel affects every cell in your body. It also affects the river of consciousness that feeds everyone. You are very important and power-ful. Your thoughts can purify the planet or contaminate it, because every thought goes into the river of consciousness. Once a thought is felt and sent out through your soul, it is available for everyone and everything.

In nature, you are fed by the vibrations of purity, life, and God, making it easier to connect with your spirit and the Infinite Mind of God. In a church or temple, you will also find vibrations of peace and love. In your own home, you can begin to build an energy of love and devotion to God by setting aside a room or area for practicing your Sacred Heart Yoga and meditations. Use the same space each time you engage in the yoga and meditation practice, and the vibrations will become purer.

This principle is also true in reverse. When you enter a place of lower vibra-tions, such as a large city or a bar, you pollute your energy field and are fed lower vibrations. This will affect your entire being, including your mental and emotional states, which in turn affects the chemical flow of your body.

How Your Thoughts Affect Your Body

Your brain is both a receiver and a transmitter of vibration. When you receive a thought, the frequency of the thought is amplified by the pineal gland and shot through the central nervous system to every nerve ending and cell in the body. The pituitary and pineal glands secrete hormones according to the vibrations they receive from the thoughts. Your thoughts and their frequencies govern your entire body chemistry.

In Sacred Heart Yoga, you hold, focus on, and embrace pure thoughts that create higher-frequency vibrations in your body. When you reach these higher frequencies, your brain begins to activate, your sacred seals begin to activate, and the kundalini flows freely.

Your thoughts become part of every cell in your body. When you embrace a thought emotionally, it is stored in the cells and becomes the mind of the body. As you embrace the higher vibrations of truth, your flesh becomes purified and vibrates at a higher frequency. Illumination then occurs in the flesh, and a radiant light emanates from within you.

Becoming a Christ, God's Ideal of Humankind
JESUS SPEAKS

First, you must have faith, believing that God is within you and that this source of power can create all things that you need to take you forward on your journey into Christhood.

Bless the Father within, and give thanks to the beloved God within you for all your good. By loving and blessing the Father within, you become the God that is within you, for whatever you focus on multiplies. In this way, you accept the truth. You experience the Father within, and what you experience becomes knowledge within you. You become God-realized, a Christ. God is then alive in every cell of your body.

As you meditate, enter into the state of Holy Communion, which is receiving the vibrations of love, wisdom, and guidance from your own divine essence. Your brain receives the frequencies of this truth through your spirit. The brain then sends pulses of these vibrations to the body through the central nervous system. Your body will begin to vibrate and even quake from these vibrations because each nerve ending is receiving the electrical shock of a high voltage of energy. This begins to ascend the density of your physical body form into light, love, and joy. As the cells receive the pulses of divine thought through energy, this divine energy projects into every cell of your body. This is created when the divine energy in the cells multiplies itself.

Each organ of your body is an amplifying center for these holy thoughts of truth. When each organ vibrates and amplifies the truth, there is great harmony in the body. You then stand and have dominion over your life, and you bring forth the Holy Spirit into creative action. The soul and the body become one force, one power, and one God. This is wholeness. You then stand as a supreme human, an all-powerful Christ.

First, you must have the desire to become the supreme, powerful human and then have a great desire to move your will into action. The greater your desire, the more powerful your will becomes, for desire is needed to add the spark of life to your will. When there is great harmony between your will and your desire, then your will springs forth, and its command is brought forth immediately into life.

The Aum

The Aum is an attempt to reproduce the sounds of creation. As you sound the Aum, you become one with the mystical tones of the universe. Mystical sounds have the ability to change the frequency of our bodies. Everything that comes into form in our dimension comes in on sound and light waves. Sound and light are one, and they work together in harmony.

In the practice of Sacred Heart Yoga, the Aum will assist you in moving the energy through the body. As you sound "Aum," you will release blockages from the body. A very pure sound can penetrate through matter, rearranging the molecules and atoms. You will become purer and clearer as you continue to practice Sacred Heart Yoga, allowing your sounding to become more effective and profound. Remember the biblical story of the walls of Jericho crumbling from the pure sounds, much like a soprano's tones can break glass.

When I first started channeling for audiences, I would go into prayer and meditation in preparation for Jesus to enter my being. He stood on my right side, waiting and asking me to sound. I am no singer and had frequently been criticized as a child for singing offkey. Instantly, I replied, "No!" to which he calmly and firmly said, "Open your mouth and sound." Again, I told him I wouldn't sing. While the audience patiently waited, I continued my resistant dialogue with Jesus. With kindness and firmness, he persisted in his requests. Finally, I agreed and opened my mouth. As I sounded, I found that the fear left my body, and my frequency began to lighten until my ego stepped aside and allowed Jesus in. Hopefully, you won't be as resistant as I was to using sound.

A nurse in one of my classes brought to my attention that sounding the Aum is a bodily release. Bodily releases occur naturally when the atoms of the body are overstressed and out of balance. The body makes the adjustments through an "arf," which may be a hiccup, sneeze, cough, belch, passing wind, and so on. This arf is an attempt to bring balance back to the body. When we sound "Aum," the same process of returning balance to the body at the atomic level occurs.

The Meaning of the Aum
A — Awakening of the God within
U — Unification with the Christ within
M — Mastery of the God I Am

The Aum Exercise

Bring your attention and awareness down to the second seal. Contract the muscles of your abdomen, pushing them toward your spine. As you do so, let the sound of the *A* come forth from within you. Feel it as it resonates in your body, tuning your cells to the sound of awakening the God (Shakti) within. Another way to awaken the God within is by singing. Jesus would sing this ancient prayer through me in order to lift my vibration: *O ma ha ne a, o tu tu ta te o,* which means, "O my God, I love you." Sing the prayer, and feel your energies come alive in you.

Now move to your third seal in the solar plexus area. Breathe in and sound out the *U*. Feel the vibrations as they move through you, bringing unification with your own Christ source. You may also say, "I unite with the Christ within me" and then sound out the *U* to experience the sensations in your third seal.

Last, bring your attention to the heart seal. Sound out the *M*. Feel the vibration in your heart center bringing the mastery to the love within so that it can be freely expressed. Remain in the heart, and reverently say the prayer, "My God, my love," three times. Now sound the *M* three more times, and notice what you are experiencing in your heart.

The Power of Spoken Word

When you speak your prayers out loud, you are practicing laya yoga. As you begin to embody the word as Jesus teaches, you will feel the thrill in your nervous system and pleasure in your cells.

The language that Jesus spoke was multilayered, alive with vibration and the life of wisdom and love. Sacred Heart Yoga follows the formula that Jesus taught in the Aramaic Lord's Prayer, which was a prayer of healing and evolution. Sacred Heart Yoga is a multilayered practice that takes the devotee deeper and deeper into self and into the essence of life that dwells within and breathes through humanity.

In Sacred Heart Yoga, you speak the prayers out loud with deeply felt sincerity, speaking from the well of emotions within. When you speak with deeply felt emotion, your spirit will begin to become alive within you. Your emotional body is the connecting link to your spiritual body.

JESUS SPEAKS

Thought is the creative vibration of life. As you speak, embrace the thought with your emotions, and bring forth your desire into the word so that the word has the energy and vibration of truth, of spirit. The moment you bring your spirit into the spoken word, the faster it shall manifest.

It is the energy in the word that gives power to the word. So as you speak, so must you become the spoken word. Become the word of God by embracing the word until every atom of your being vibrates with the energy of the word. Then you are the living word of God. You are then in the state of love.

You will find that when the word is filled with the emotion of love, you can move into the all-loving substance of God, and you can manifest all things from the substance through your divine thoughts. When this concept is realized and understood, you serve the God of your being, and your service is joyful.

You are ruler in your domain, and you will begin to experience having dominion over your life. You will live God's will for you, and you will then experience heaven.

You will use these principles throughout your Sacred Heart Yoga practice. You will learn and understand the awe, wonder, and power of the spoken word. You will begin to feel yourself become the substance of God. You will feel pleasure, light, and timelessness, and you will know that all things are possible with God.

The Awe of Becoming the Spoken Word

In 1994, I was leading a workshop to activate the sacred seals for a Michigan group. We had rented a retreat house in the country on a lake (because this kind of work is best suited to a pure atmosphere in nature).

While lying on the floor with my arms outstretched from the shoulders, palms facing up, I was lost in God's love. I had become one with the substance of God and was saying the attunement, or prayer, for activation.

When I was complete and had come back to this dimension, I saw that there were cracks in the palms of my hands, just as if they had been sliced with a very fine razor, and there was a cross design on each hand. The bleeding lasted about four hours. Today, there are still crosses where my palms bled. I was told that stigmata had occurred in my palms while in this state of oneness with the divine.

CHAPTER **8**

Attunements

In speaking your prayers of devotion, you practice laya yoga. Prayers and mantras are the practice of laya yoga. The result of your heartfelt devotion and commitment to the practice of Sacred Heart Yoga brings knowledge, or gnana yoga. In gnana yoga, you become so connected to the indwelling wisdom and knowledge that it vibrates through you, resulting in you suddenly realizing the truth. Knowledge and self-realization are attained.

With each asana, you say a prayer. These prayers are designed to invoke the divine within. They must be filled with your life essence and a moving power to bring forth the desired result. The prayers are directly and energetically linked to the sacred seals and energy system of the body.

An attunement is not an affirmation. Attunements are mantras, the language of God, which is vibration and energy. As you speak with truth, you become the vibration of God. You are like a tuning fork, attuning yourself to the words you are speaking. You are becoming the frequency of these words. You must become the vibration of the words of love and truth. Once you do, you are the living word, and it shall manifest with no effort on your part.

Jesus shared the spiritual wisdom of prayers with me in the four teachings that follow.

FIRST TEACHING FROM JESUS
When you hold the truth in your consciousness, you become the living word of God. You will then learn that Spirit is the fulfillment of the need.

In speaking the prayers in Sacred Heart Yoga, you become completely focused in the moment and devoted to the Divine in movement and prayer. You have given God your complete being. As you fully and completely give yourself to God, you become the vibration of the words that you are speaking. Once you have become the vibration of the words, they become alive with God's life and will manifest.

SECOND TEACHING FROM JESUS

When you hold the vibration of God in your being, you build your inner world as you choose. God is the fullness of all good.

You will learn that when you feel in need, it is because of a sense of lack or emptiness. Bring your need to the God within, and become filled with energy, love, wisdom, or whatever is needed.

While moving into the ancient postures and speaking the prayers aloud, focus on and feel from deep in your heart and soul what you are saying to become the vibration of God. Your outer world is a reflection of your inner life, for in that moment of devotion, you consciously choose to be dedicated to your God. In turn, God fills your world with good.

THIRD TEACHING FROM JESUS

You will begin to understand the spiritual truth of your prayers. Then you will begin to feel the atmosphere of the light of God around you and within you. You will also begin to understand and feel that the Father and you are one. As you practice Sacred Heart Yoga, your vibrations will continue to quicken, and you will move into states of ecstasy and bliss. Your body and the atmosphere around it will be filled with light. You will feel as if you are in another state of consciousness, bathed in beautiful energy. It is the Father within consuming you.

FOURTH TEACHING FROM JESUS

As you express the words, let love flow through you. When love flows through your consciousness, your cells respond and are caressed by it. The flesh becomes radiant, renewed, purified, and quickened in its vibrations. The I Am is expressed through the flesh, the mind becomes enlightened, and the soul becomes educated. The body becomes obedient to the spirit and expresses spirit through it.

Putting into words my experience of what it feels like to have God caress me with love is very difficult. Being pleasured and bathed with God's love is beyond any human experience I ever had. Also, this is not a one-time experience. It occurs each time that I allow love to flow through my consciousness, and my physical cell body responds. I feel intoxicated with love, lost in love, as it consumes every cell in my body — bringing pleasure to the body and soothing my heart and emotions. I am suspended in a timeless love that is so complete that I cannot think of anything that I want or need. In that moment, I have everything.

Sacred Heart Yoga Prayer

Beloved Father,
I devote this practice this day
to the evolution of my soul and
to the fulfillment of my destiny in service to the One,
and I allow myself to be purified
as I rejoice in the kingdom of heaven
and in the love of God.
I give thanks for this blessing and
for these moments that I share with my body
and my spirit in onement.
And so it is. Amen.

CHAPTER 9

Service to the God Within

This phase of Sacred Heart Yoga begins with karma yoga, the yoga of service, and also includes laya yoga and gnana yoga. In this practice, you will ask the divine essence within you how you can personally serve life and your unfoldment. This question is your prayer connected to practicing laya yoga. The information or guidance received is knowledge. This knowledge is gnana yoga.

When Jesus taught me about serving God within, he gave me one lesson daily. Some lessons were repeated for several days, or even months, until I understood the meaning and how to use this wisdom to realize my oneness with the Father/ Mother God within.

Jesus says, "It is your willingness to serve God that opens the doorway within to the kingdom of God's wealth." These are beautiful words, but what do they mean in everyday life? I learned to listen to myself and observe my thoughts in relation to this concept of serving God. Just the word "service" triggered a negative response in my mind and body. I will share how I overcame this negative response to fully and joyfully embrace serving God.

Service Exercise

Read Jesus's words — "It is your willingness to serve God that opens the doorway within to the kingdom of God's wealth" — and then close your eyes. Notice how your body responds to this concept of service. What does your mind chatter say? Watch your thoughts as if you are viewing a TV screen. Become an observer of your mind chatter.

Write below how your body responded to the concept of service.

_____

_____

What thoughts came to you about this concept?

_____

_____

_____

_____

What were your feelings about service to God?

_____

_____

If you find any doubt, confusion, or resistance to living in service to God, then speak to this part of yourself out loud. Give yourself guidance and encouragement as if you were speaking to a friend or your inner child. This may take more than one conversation, depending how much resistance there is. Once this resistant aspect of you chooses to join in your service to God, you will find that you feel more congruent within yourself. You will move at a much more rapid pace into alignment with God's will for you. This occurs because your soul has begun to return home to the Father's house and its original purpose.

Each day, as you continue to ask for your service, you will find your life blessed with goodness. Life will become effortless, and you'll feel your oneness with the God within growing. The Father within becomes your partner in life. You are no longer alone but are now supported in life by the divine Source within.

Giving and Receiving through Service

"The servant lives outside of the Father's house. The servant seeks to attain entrance into the Father's house," Jesus said. We can attain all things by looking within ourselves and living in the kingdom, in the Father/Mother God's house. We live outside of the Father's house when we think we are alone. The ego tries to make it all happen independently, so then we come from need. The need may be to achieve material possessions, to feel important, or to be acknowledged by others. When we come from need, we project ourselves into life. Jesus would tell me, "There is no need to project yourself. Know that you are the truth of God. You are not here to receive applause or to be greater than another. You are here to serve the Father within you." This always brought me back into alignment, which helped me surrender my need to receive from outside of me. I could once again bring my focus back to my service to God in that moment.

This takes conscious commitment and practice. So be patient with yourself. You are learning a new way of living, and the ego personality self is dissolving. The old behavior patterns begin to break up and dissipate. Your addictions will begin to fall away one by one. All this is done in service to the God within.

As you continue to ask God for your service, you will begin receiving divine messages of truth. Through this process, you will find that you move very rapidly through the darkness, cleansing and purifying your mind, body, and soul, because you are working at the atomic level of your being, re-creating your cells to radiate and vibrate the truth. The body is becoming clearer, a clearer channel for the God of your being.

We begin our Sacred Heart Yoga by asking the God within for our service. In this way, we begin to know God's will for us. Jesus would say to me, "God knows and the human thinks (the ego)." In my experience, service is always meant to evolve or develop myself. It may simply be to give myself what I need, to know something, to acknowledge that I am loved, or to be kind to myself. You may ask, for example, to rest to remain in balance, know all is in divine order, accept that you are loved, or keep walking forward on your path. This practice puts me on my path of truth and purpose.

Jesus taught me that as we serve God, he in turn serves us even more so. This is the law of giving and receiving. You begin to know that the God within will serve you, and this is a very secure feeling. You know you can rely on God for your needs. God becomes your partner and greatest friend in life.

As you practice living in service to God, your wants will greatly diminish because you will be filled with such love. This leaves you feeling lighter, freer, safer, and more complete.

Choosing God
JESUS SPEAKS

There is but one choice, one purpose, one truth, and one science. First, you must choose God. Then have it be your purpose to serve God. As you serve God, he in turn serves you even greater. You become as God is, and you then can express God's goodness and grace through you. Humankind is the Christ of God, the ideal of God, created in God's image and likeness. You must have the intention to be and live the truth of God, for in this way you live the true science of life. You will become God's ideal man, God's ideal woman, a Christ. Rejoice in this journey home to the beloved Father within you.

When I began to look at these powerful statements and realize what they meant, I was overwhelmed with the changes I would have to make in my life to fulfill this and live the true science of life. I wasn't sure I was ready to surrender so much of my ego to God. So, little by little, I began to surrender my old ways of life. As I became more comfortable with the process of surrendering my ego, I began to feel the truth of who I am inside, no longer so fearful and self-conscious. I couldn't wait to choose God in other areas of my life. I decided to choose God instead of choosing to get attention from outside of me. I asked God for help in prayer.

My Prayer

Beloved Father, I love you, and I need you to help me overcome my need for attention from the world around me.

I'm tired of trying to please the world.

I truly desire to live for you and please you, beloved Father.

Once I made the choice to live for God, I became very conscious of how I wanted and needed attention from others. The following is an example of how I began to notice different aspects of my personality.

In classes at my health club, I normally would be totally absorbed in my own yoga practice. I do yoga with my eyes closed, which takes me into bliss. As I opened my eyes one day, I became aware of my thoughts and fears of being judged by others in the class. I felt different from them because I had all of this blissful energy moving through my body. Many of the others were new to yoga and came for the exercise. They were not on a spiritual path and certainly not aware of the divine energy within them. Ten or fifteen minutes after this thought, I noticed a different aspect of myself — a part of me that felt proud of being so spiritually advanced. As you can see, I was trapped in fear and pride, part of me feeling fearful of being judged because I was different and another aspect feeling proud of my perceived advanced spirituality.

Each time one of these unhealed, unenlightened aspects of me would raise her head, I would ask her to come Home and choose God. I would tell her that God is the source of her good and that she could and would receive what she needed from the God within. This process of lovingly teaching and guiding the unhealed parts of myself continued for about one month. I was teaching myself a new truth and also developing discipline as I guided myself back from the outside to the God within. One day, I felt something new inside: These aspects of self were receiving from within. I felt filled and complete with no desire to receive attention from the world around me. I no longer cared what the world thought of me. I was free. My posture changed, my shoulders opened, and I could carry myself with love and certainty, for I was living the truth and serving God, not those around me.

As I Serve God, I Serve Myself

In March 1999 I came to the realization that this work continually unfolds within me. That is what makes my life and this work so exciting. As I use these simple truths, I continue to grow, expand, purify, and ascend to the next level of understanding and truth. I realized that as I serve God, I serve myself.

This is how I arrived at my realization. One morning, I woke up feeling extremely tired. I had been battling a low-grade infection with aches, fevers, and a sore throat. The symptoms came and went. On this morning, I just wanted to sleep. The phone woke me at 8AM, a time when I'm usually up and active, but I wanted to roll over and go back to sleep. I had planned to go to my health club and participate in a body building class and then swim and work on this book. I've trained myself to speak to God as soon as I'm conscious, and I asked God, "How may I serve you today? Is it in service for me to rest in bed or to go to the club?" The answer: "Go to the club. You will find joy and inspiration there." I then pulled myself out of bed and off I went.

The class was just what my body wanted, even though it was still tired and aching. Then at the pool, I rested in the sun for half an hour before going into the water. As I jumped into the pool, I felt my entire being shift, and joy began to fill every cell until I felt effervescent in my entire being. I swam and played until I was complete. When I went back to the pool lounge, there were no aches or other symptoms left in my body. As I began to work on the book, I immediately felt filled with creativity and inspiration. A plan for my work unfolded with each detail just spilling out of me. I was so high on life that I could hardly contain my joy.

As I started to review this chapter on service, the little girl that is my ego, my unhealed self who hangs out in fear, said, "As I serve God, I serve myself." All the fear left, and joy and exultation filled my being. The vibration of my entire body had risen above the frequency of my aches, sore throat, and fever, and I was healed in that moment. I realized the truth through my experience of following my service for the day. This was an experience of physical, mental, and emotional healing. God wants the highest good for me. On the other hand, my ego, or unhealed self, is always trying to figure out what to do and how to do it. Usually, it comes up with negative thoughts. By following my service, I moved right through my ego to my divine self, which is filled with wisdom and creativity. Now I know exactly what to do and how to do it. My next step is to take action and follow through with my plan.

Exercise: Take a moment to go inside and see where you are ready to choose God. Maybe it is in relationships or maybe in your health, diet, or job. It can be in any area of your life.

TEACHING FROM JESUS
You must have the intention to be and live the truth of God, for in this way, you live the true science of life.

Once you find one part of you that is ready to change, say a prayer of intention to choose God and to serve God. Write a clear and concise prayer below, and then speak it out loud into the universe. In this way, you gather the forces of the universe to support your intention, and so it shall be.

_____

_____

_____

As you begin to look inside and observe yourself, you may become more conscious of your patterns, addictions, and old ways of living. Don't make yourself feel wrong for these things. Have the unhealed self choose God in the moment you notice the behaviors or hear the limited thoughts. You must be consistent and committed in order to heal. This is a very intentional practice of working with the unhealed self. With continued practice, one day you will be free to live the truth of God. I celebrate your life and freedom with you.

Meditation in Preparation for Service

We meditate to open ourselves to receive this divine service. To exercise this, sit in sukhasana (cross-legged) or half lotus position with your hands on your knees, palms open and facing upward.

Imagine that you have a magic wand in your right hand. Raise your right hand in front of your face. Begin to sweep your auric field, bringing the wand around and downward to the right knee and then over to the left knee and finally back upward to your head. This cuts the cords that attach you to others. As you make this sweeping movement, say this prayer, "I clear my energy field of anyone standing within it. I bless them and send them to the light."

Now place your right hand on your third chakra, and listen to the God within you. Then say, "Beloved God, how may I serve you?" As you quietly await a response, information may come to you in a sense of knowing. You may hear a voice, or a thought may become present in your mind. This information is brief and to the point. Be patient, and remain open to the possibility that your God knows, and you will receive the correct information.

You may choose to write your service down below or in a notebook. Frequently, when I receive information from my God, it is clear and vivid in the moment and then begins to fade within a few minutes, much like a dream, and I can't recall the details. So I have learned the value of writing my service.

_____

_____

_____

_____

You must trust this information and be willing to act on it, putting it into motion in your world. This is the way to master yourself and change your life experiences and circumstances. You will find that your desire to serve God will continue to expand, and you will have a greater purpose to live life.

TEACHING FROM JESUS

When you are serving God, your soul releases power and love into life.

How to Use Intentions

After surrendering to service, the second step in Sacred Heart Yoga is to take the knowledge you received about your service and make it your intention. This knowledge is gnana yoga. Whatever information or knowledge you received while asking for your service from the God within is made into a statement of intention. This puts the knowledge into action. It may simply be one word. Let's say your service is to forgive. You would stand and make a statement: "It is my intention to forgive." When you stand and speak your intention, you are making a commitment to yourself and the God within. You are living in alignment with your highest good. It is through your thoughts, deeds, and actions that you live in alignment with God's will for you. As you speak your intentions, you engage in laya yoga and begin the process of transforming the ego and compulsive behavior patterns.

The ego will continue to dissolve its need for control as you begin to rely on God more and more. When you speak your intentions from your service, it sets change in motion. You begin to heal your mind, body, and emotions. The energy field will begin to clear, and you will become more as God is. The divinity within will begin to dissolve the old ways of thinking, acting, and feeling as you take these high intentions into the Sacred Heart Yoga practice.

The intentions of your thoughts can change your perceptions, which will change your experience. Put forth your intentions to receive the truth. When you put forth your intentions in the spoken word, they can change time, erase distance, and affect all things both seen and unseen.

The purpose of speaking intentions is to become the living word of God, manifesting the word. As you speak your intention, the energy leaves your body, transmitting it to the universe. You feel this in waves of energy leaving you, and you know, in that moment, that it is done. Then you have become the living word of God, and the word shall manifest. As you continue to surrender the ego's old patterns, you become clearer and more powerful, and you will manifest more quickly.

The process of speaking your intentions leads you into the third stage of Sacred Heart Yoga, which is mastery. Mastery is the experience of manifesting your intention. You will have mastered your thoughts, your emotions, and your body. Your body will then respond to your spirit. Jesus would tell me, "Let your spirit have full sway in your body." That is why you may experience spontaneous movements in the body as you practice the yoga: Your spirit is moving you. In that moment, body and soul become one force, and as one force, you manifest. You are one, no longer split into fragments.

I will share with you how I have taken my own intentions and raised them to the next level where I experience instant transformation. I allow the wounded part of myself (the fearful or resistant ego self) to speak the intention. This is the part of me that needs to be healed. My ego, in that moment, surrenders to God's will, or divine plan; as the fear or resistance is dissolved, my energy becomes heightened, and I am a reborn being. My weakness becomes my strength, and I am filled with love and power.

When you stand and speak your intentions, you may experience your body begin to vibrate or a breath spontaneously move through you. You are raising your vibration, consciously choosing a new way — a new life, the life of God, union with the Divine. In this process of speaking intentions aloud, you implant this vibration into the soul, manifesting it. You are working in partnership with the Divine. The grace of God will be upon you. In my classes, when students sincerely speak their intentions from the heart and soul, waves of energy travel throughout the room from their bodies, causing tingles and shivers. This is a sign that the intention is on its way to manifestation.

JESUS SPEAKS

True power is in the truth of God. Speak the words of truth and love, and let yourself be filled with your own vibrations of love and light. Intentions bring you into oneness with the Father within, for in this way you begin to live a life of focus, a life of goodness. You engage your divine spirit, and you begin to allow this divine power that is within you to live your life, letting go of the needs of the ego. You begin to live the truth of your divine self, which is love, grace, and God-power.

Your deeds, your actions, become pure. Honor returns to you, and then you are living your Christ self. The life that you live becomes dedicated to the God within. You live a life of devotion to God by your deeds, actions, and the thoughts that you hold. Your intention creates movement forward. You are consciously choosing to live in alignment to God's will for you.

Stand and speak your intentions into the universal river of consciousness. By having an intention and speaking it, you begin to focus on the truth and on love, and this tames your animal soul. With your intentions, you take control of your life and return home to the beloved Father within you.

As you put forth your intentions, they will manifest for you. This manifestation will become swifter and swifter as your power grows. I salute the Christ of your being — God's ideal woman, God's ideal man.

CHAPTER 10

Devotion:
the First Stage of Surrender

The first stage of surrender postures and prayers is extremely significant because the results you receive from Sacred Heart Yoga depend on your union with the indwelling presence. This union is created through devotion, which is bhakti yoga. It will purify your soul and bring peace to your heart. Your relationship with the divine female and divine male aspects of self begins with devotional bhakti yoga. Through your love, you fuse together the human and divine within you. The dance of tantra begins. Each time you practice Sacred Heart Yoga, your relationship with the divine female and divine male grows stronger and more intense. Then the kundalini will begin its movement up the spine, and it will bring tingling sensations to the nervous system. You may feel warmth as the heat intensifies within you. Laya yoga and hatha yoga are practiced as part of this powerful series of devotional surrender asanas.

Jesus spoke in Aramaic, a multilayered language. In Aramaic, the word for devotion was "surrender." To be devoted to the Divine meant to surrender to the Divine. There was no other way.

The first stage of surrender captivates your entire being, bringing all the seals and chakras into alignment to God's life. This is the life of love and light that is within you. The asanas in this series develop your relationship with the God within through devotional love. You develop a love that is based on trust. This stage of surrender is reached through devotion to the Mother/Father God within. Deep in the soul is the desire to love God. It is the forgotten song we wish to sing.

Sacred Heart Yoga leads you into a deep state of devotion to the God within. You will learn to focus the mind on devotional prayers. As you focus on the prayer or the thought, you learn to master the mind by stilling the chatter. In this way, you learn to control your thoughts and break free from the undisciplined mind. Then you will feel your love for God as you speak the prayer aloud. This energy of love begins to multiply within your body, which feels light, alive, tingly, and vital. You may even begin to feel orgasmic pleasure as you surrender to God's love for you.

Your body will be in devotion through ancient movements and mystical sounds. In this way, your entire being is in devotion — mind, emotions, and body. As you deeply surrender to the energy of God, you begin to allow God to have full sway in your body. Then you begin to become as God is. Jesus would tell me, "Whatever you focus on multiplies. By loving and blessing the Father within, you become the God that is within you."

Your ego must yield to the pleasure of God moving through your body. As you devote your entire being to loving God, you enter the state of surrender. The God within begins to expand, and the energy of your own divinity multiplies. Your body becomes obedient to your spirit as the sacred energy moves through it, bringing it into the natural movements of surrender where your head begins to move back and your chest moves upward, creating an arch in your spine behind the heart seal. It may feel as though you are pinned back by the energy and unable to move. Do not be frightened, and allow these movements without trying to control them. The God within will move and live through you. You then have begun to manifest oneness with God in the physical form. To enter this state of oneness, you must have surrendered to the sacred energy of your God within. This is the natural evolution of your divine being coming to life, the life within.

The key to developing a body that is obedient to spirit is devotion. Jesus would tell me, "Your devotion to God must be all-encompassing. You must live the life of truth, the life of devotion to God and not to the material world. Then and only then are you the heir to your Father's kingdom."

You attain your experience of oneness as you deeply feel your love of God. When you speak your attunements, your prayers, feel each word. When you feel your love, you are in the process of becoming the living word of God. This is the process of attuning yourself to the vibration of the words of love that you speak. As you do so, you become the vibration of the words.

The Power of Devotion

Jesus explained the power of devotion to me in October 1998 in this way:

When you praise, bless, and worship the God within, you bring forth the power and love of God. Then this power and love of God emanates from within you. The vibrations of God flow through you and around you. You envelop all with the vibrations of God.

Through your devotion to God, you become the vibration of God, the light of God. Then and only then do you have the power to conduct the forces of the universe. You have become one with the light of God and the forces of the universe. There is no difference between you and God. You have become the same. You have become a spiritual being, not a material being; therefore, you have the power to conduct and direct the light of God outside of you as well as within you, for in that moment, you are one with the light. If you love God with all of your being, it soon becomes a habit: It is your daily life and existence. You then have brought forth your divinity. As long as you stay true to the vibrations of God, you will never know strife nor will you perish.

When you unite with the God within, you can conquer all things. The power is drawn to you and generated within your body, and it is sent forth to accomplish whatever you direct it to bring forth. This is God living through you, emanating the force of good through you. When you send the Father before you to prepare your way, you are with God, and the Father penetrates all things. Together you conquer your life. Your life becomes godly, godlike, good. You and the God within have become one force sent forth to manifest.

In my early years with Jesus, I was in such disbelief. This all sounded so easy. With Jesus coaching me, I learned how to send the Father before me. Each morning before getting out of bed, he would have me send the Father before me to accomplish whatever I needed. To my surprise, it worked! Each time, as I expand and manifest all that I need, I move to the next state in my own development. However, there will always be unknown challenges. I have been asked to do things I've never done before, and I still face my own doubts, fears, and unworthiness. But I try to dissolve my walls of fear and doubt.

While I was living on the Big Island of Hawaii, Jesus suggested I make a video of Sacred Heart Yoga. Instantly I replied, "I'd love to, but where am I going to get the thousands for this project?" Jesus instructed me to send the Father before me, which I did. Amazingly it worked. One evening while teaching my weekly yoga class in the small town of Hawi, the northernmost point on the island, a man named David entered, carrying a video camera. David asked if he could videotape our Sacred Heart Yoga class. His project was a community program advertising Hawi spiritual and cultural events. That class was taught by candlelight, so I did not feel that it was appropriate to film. However, I invited David to join us for the class, which he did.

A few days later, we met for lunch, and he agreed to film and produce my Sacred Heart Yoga video. When we discussed the cost, his answer was heavenly. David agreed to gift the video to me in support of my work. The Father within had responded once again.

With this example in mind, I invite you to send the Father before you in your life. Here is the prayer Jesus taught me: "Beloved Father, go before me, and prepare the way for _____" (state specifically what you need). The benefits of the first stage of surrender are very incredible. The greatest is entering into oneness with the God within you. This is the love for which we have all been waiting.

As you develop this state of oneness, God will begin to think your thoughts and speak profound truth and wisdom through you as you. In this state of love, hormones are released from the pituitary and pineal glands. You will feel younger and excited to be alive. You will develop the power to manifest as you create this union with the divine within. Your divine essence will respond to your desires and your requests. Jesus states it this way: "When you give your life to the Father/Mother within — the source of your true love, wisdom, and power — you enter the unknown state of oneness. You must surrender to God to know God. Once you have reached the state of surrendering to God, the divine energy of God will move through you as you."

You will begin to experience the presence of God within as you continue with your practice of Sacred Heart Yoga and truly begin to surrender. This will allow you to surrender even more. You come to know God through your experience of the presence within. You will feel this presence within and all around you as love and as pleasure. The energy and essence of the divine forces of love will intoxicate you and bring you into the state of bliss and oneness. This Shakti, or Holy Spirit, energy moves through your body and heals.

You will find that you lose interest in the material world as you deeply surrender. Jesus told me that, "When you surrender completely to God, you live in the world but not of it. You will not be involved in worldly activities, but only those that the Father/Mother guides you to participate in."

Old patterns and needs will fall away. Even your addictions will begin to dissolve one by one, naturally, effortlessly. When I began this journey with Sacred Heart Yoga and Jesus, I was addicted to cigarettes. I had been smoking since I was a teenager. Slowly, I began to smoke less and less until one day I realized I would never smoke again. This process took two years. I was not even trying to quit smoking. Quitting simply occurred as I began to hold more light in my physical body. The cigarettes and I were not of the same frequency. The desire to smoke was gone. I desired to feed my body food and other substances of lighter frequencies.

The Divine Flow of Prayers in the First Series of Surrender

The prayers in the first series of surrender create a divine flow of energy that moves through your entire being. The flow of postures, prayers, and mystical tones prepares you for activation of the sacred seals.

1. Begin to speak prayers of love and devotion to the Mother/Father within. These devotional prayers and feelings of love bring us into a state of oneness with God.

2. The flow of prayers moves to the next octave in which you give your life to God. As you do, you begin to feel the life of God within. Separation no longer exists.

3. As you continue the prayers, your vibration quickens. Then you move into trusting God with your life. As you trust, God will begin to heal the betrayals, disappointments, abandonments, and rejections you have experienced in your life and relationships. Your vibration will quicken even more, purifying at a cellular level.

The First Series of Surrender Postures

The right side of the body is our male energy, also known as positive, or electrical, energy. The left side is our female energy, also known as negative, or magnetic, energy. In some cultures, the male and female energy is referred to as yang and yin, respectively. In Sacred Heart Yoga, we refer to the male side as the beloved Father and the female side as the beloved Mother. The Father energy is the light of God, holding our wisdom, guidance, strength, courage, and protection. The Mother energy is the love of God, holding our compassion, intuition, gentleness, kindness, and nurturing qualities.

Always begin the leg postures with the right leg, as this works in harmony with the natural flow of energy in the physical body. Working in opposition to the energy in the ascending colon may create a blockage.

Lie on your back with legs fully extended, arms at sides and the palms of your hands facing upward. Relax. Take a moment to let your body blend into the mat, consciously letting go. Breathe deeply into your body, and sound out the ancient sound of "Aum," letting go of any old thoughts, worries, and doubts.

Guidelines for Speaking the Prayers

Each time you lie down to begin Sacred Heart Yoga, you speak directly from your heart to the God within. The prayers must be in the moment, and they must be real. The prayers I offer as examples were the prayers I used at the time of writing. If you desire to generate your own prayers, use the following guidelines:

- Speak the love that is in your heart to the Father (right side) and the Mother (left side).
- Tell the Father and Mother what is going on in your life. Have a personal conversation.
- Share yourself with your divine essence. Tell the Mother and Father your challenges, your problems, your fears, your worries, and your joys — whatever is there. Cry your tears, and feel your feelings. Let the magic of transformation occur.
- In this humble, honest prayer, you enter the sacred heart, where the answer and love you need exist.

Bring the right knee to the chest, embracing it with the arms and pulling it as close to your body as you can on the outbreath. Keep your shoulders relaxed (fig.1).

In this way, you open the first sacred seal and chakra, surrendering to the divinity within.

Once in position, take a moment to feel your love for the Father within. Let this love for God fill you. Become completely focused and devoted to your love for the Father. Nothing else exists in this moment but your love for God. Speak the prayer aloud and sound out the Aum. The pattern of speaking a prayer and sounding the Aum continues in each asana.

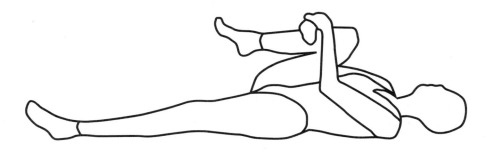

Figure 1

PRAYER
Beloved Father, I love you.
I love you with all of my heart, with all of my mind,
and with all of my strength.
Aum.

Breathe in; and as you exhale, bring your knee even closer into your body, surrendering a bit more into the posture. Once again, sound out the Aum.

Place your left hand on the right foot, gently guiding the foot over to the left thigh; let the right knee fall to the floor. Allow the weight of your knee to take it toward the floor. Bring the right arm above your head, extending it fully and elongating the right side of your body (fig.2).

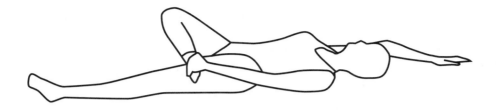

Figure 2

PRAYER
I willingly surrender.
I surrender to the will of God for me,
and I allow myself to move forward in truth
and in love, serving you.
Aum.

Surrender as you open your hip joint and pelvic area, opening the first and second seals. Feel your willingness to serve God and your willingness to surrender. Let yourself open to this concept. Let the body open to the energy of surrender and service.

Bring your right hand down and grasp the right foot. Bend the knee and pull the foot up flexing the foot. Your knee will gently move closer to your head. Extend the left arm above your head, pointing the left toes and stretching your left arm and hand (fig. 3).

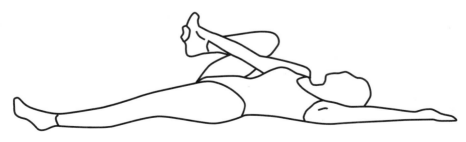

Figure 3

PRAYER
I am your child.
I come to you in pureness
and in vulnerability.
I open my heart to love you.
I open my mind to hear your wisdom.
I open my body to feel you.
Aum.

Feel your vulnerability. Open to it, knowing you are safe in God's loving arms. Remember, the Father is within you, and you are within the Father.

Raise the right foot to the heavens, and then gently pull down with the right hand so that the knee moves closer and closer toward the earth, opening the hip and groin areas (fig. 4), letting go.

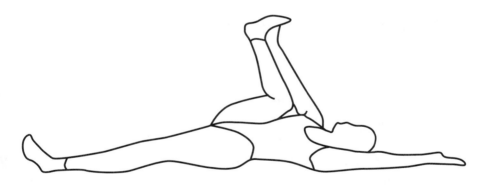

Figure 4

PRAYER
Beloved Father,
I surrender to you.
Consume me with your love,
and heal me.
Aum.

Take a moment to feel the energy of the Father's love as it consumes and heals you, and give thanks.

Let go of your foot, allowing the foot to begin to rise upward. Extend the arms out from your shoulders, palms facing up. Slowly allow the leg to fall open and downward to the right. Roll the foot to the right as the inner thigh opens (fig. 5).

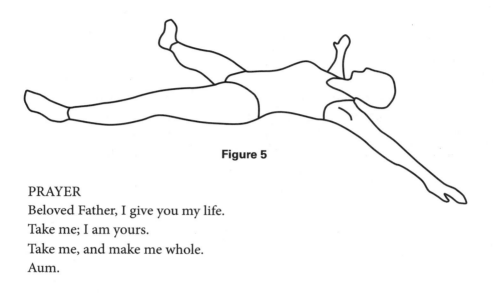

Figure 5

PRAYER
Beloved Father, I give you my life.
Take me; I am yours.
Take me, and make me whole.
Aum.

Feel yourself yielding to the Father. Open the heart as you have never opened it before. Turn your head to the right, keeping the right shoulder on the mat. Let the right leg cross over the body, letting the weight of the leg open the spine as you twist, allowing the vertebrae in your back to open (fig. 6). Surrender, and let bliss flow freely through you.

Now arch your back, and breathe into the heart seal, keeping the right shoulder on the ground. Open to life, to joy, and to love (fig. 6).

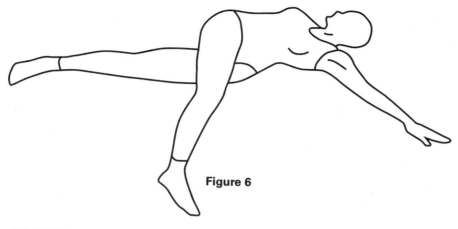

Figure 6

PRAYER
I thank you, Father. I love you, Father,
and I love myself. I thank myself
for being in this moment,
surrendering and realizing the truth of my being.
Aum.

Return the leg back to center, and allow it to come down on the mat. Bring the arms back down to the sides, palms facing upward. Feel the energy in the right side of your body. As you continue to lie basking and bathing in God's love, say a prayer of thanksgiving.

PRAYER
Beloved God, I give thanks
for this moment of now
and for living in oneness with you,
serving you and letting you live through me.
Amen, amen, amen.

Bring the left knee to the chest, embracing it with your arms and pulling it close to the body. Keep the shoulders relaxed (fig. 7). In this way, you open the first seal, preparing to surrender into the divinity within.

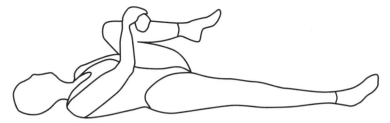

Figure 7

PRAYER
Beloved Mother, I love you.
I thank you for your
nurturing love.
Aum.

Feel the Mother's love for you. Accept that this love is renewing and restoring your body to its perfection.

Place the right hand on your left foot. Gently guide the foot over to the right thigh, letting the knee fall to the ground. Allow the weight of your knee to take it toward the mat. Extend the left arm above your head, elongating the left side of your body (fig. 8).

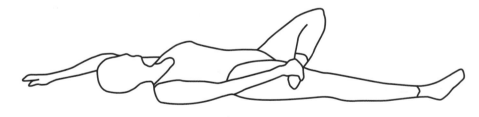

Figure 8

PRAYER
I surrender to your kindness,
beloved Mother.
I no longer resist you.
I let your love
come forth from within me.
Aum.

The Mother's love can heal your broken heart. She can heal the emotion of pain. Open yourself to receive her gift of loving kindness.

Bring your left hand down, and grasp the left foot. Bend the left knee and pull up on the foot, flexing the foot. Your knee will gently move closer to your head. Extend the right arm above the head. Point the right toes, and extend the right arm and hand (fig. 9).

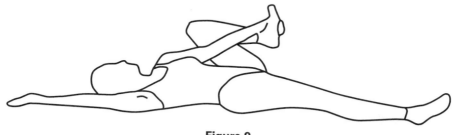

Figure 9

PRAYER
Beloved Mother, I love you,
and I need you.
I am your child.
I devote myself to you
in this moment.
Aum.

Feel your devotion and love for the Mother within. Focus your mind on your love for her. Raise the left foot to the heavens. Gently pull down with your left hand so that the knee moves closer and closer toward the mat, opening the hip and groin areas (fig. 10), letting go.

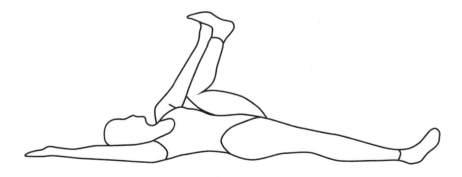

Figure 10

PRAYER
I surrender my mind.
I surrender my heart.
I surrender my body to you.
Beloved Mother, I love you with
all that I am in this moment.
Aum.

Feel the love that is offered to you in this moment. Allow yourself to receive more fully than ever before. As you serve the Mother, she serves you even greater.

Let go of your foot, allowing it to begin to rise upward. Extend your arms out from your shoulders, palms facing up. Now let the leg fall open and downward to the left. Roll the foot to the left as the inner thigh opens (fig. 11). Feel your vulnerability, remembering that you are safe in God's love.

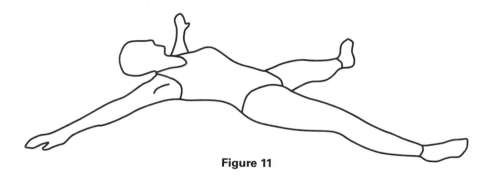

Figure 11

PRAYER
I give my life to you,
fully and completely, Mother,
in this moment and forever.
I am here to serve you,
and I love you now and forever.
Aum.

As you give your life to the Mother, you become the life of the Mother. She will begin to love through you, as you.

Turn your head to the left. Keep the left shoulder on the mat. Let the left leg cross over the body, and allow the weight of the leg to open your spine as you twist (fig. 12). Surrender to the energy of love, allowing it to flow freely within. Now arch your back, breathe into the heart seal, and keep the left shoulder on the mat. Open your heart, mind, and body to be filled with love.

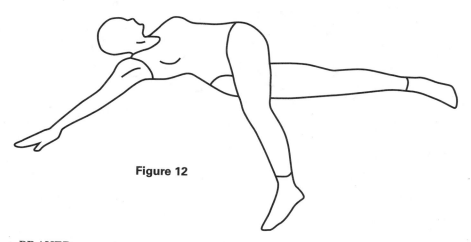

Figure 12

PRAYER
I thank you, Mother. I love you, Mother,
and I love myself. I thank myself
for allowing me to be in this moment,
surrendering and realizing
the truth of my being.
Aum.

Return the leg to center, allowing it to come back down to the mat. Bring your arms back down to the sides, palms facing upward. Feel the energy in the left side of the body.

Continuing on, you will now work with both legs. This series of asanas develops the main channel of light that runs up your spine. These asanas are designed to open the lower back, the second seal, which is the seal of relationships, so you will develop your relationship with the God of your being. The divinity of the second seal is developed through trust, and these prayers are designed to bring you into a state of trust. Continue with your own heartfelt prayers. Trust that you will be transformed.

Bend both knees, pulling them into the chest (fig. 13), embracing them with love, and gently pull them even closer to your heart as you exhale.

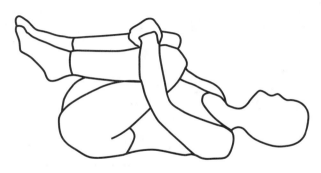

Figure 13

PRAYER
I trust you with my life,
beloved God.
I trust you.
Aum.

Begin to become aware of your state of being, and question your resistance to trusting God with your life.

Place the soles of your feet together. Bring your hands inside the knees, and take hold of the feet with your hands, interlacing the fingers. Just allow your knees to fall open as you press the soles of the feet together (fig. 14). This creates a pyramid over the first sacred seal.

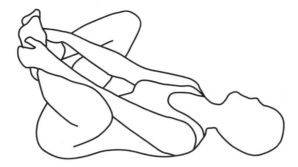

Figure 14

PRAYER
Beloved God,
you are within me, and
I am safe in your love and light.
Aum.

Let yourself begin to sink into the feeling of safety with the God within.

Part the feet and hands; continue to grasp the feet. Pull up on the bottoms of your feet so that the knees move toward your shoulders (fig. 15).

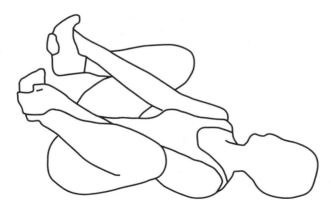

Figure 15

PRAYER
I trust you,
my beloved God,
to bring me the love that I need to heal,
to grow, and to be nourished
in this dimension.
Aum.

Allow the energy of safety to fill you. Let the muscles in your back relax. Feel your spine soften as you surrender.

Lift your feet toward the heavens. As you exhale, pull down on your feet, bending the knees and bringing them closer to the earth (fig. 16).

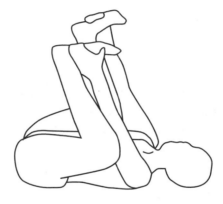

Figure 16

PRAYER
I surrender now.
It is safe to surrender to you,
for I am safe in your love and light.
I trust you to lead me home.
Aum.

This is the greatest opening in the lower back. Feel your second seal opening as you trust more deeply.

Extend your arms from the shoulders, palms facing downward. Let the knees fall to the right as your head moves to the left (fig. 17). Keep the left shoulder on the mat.

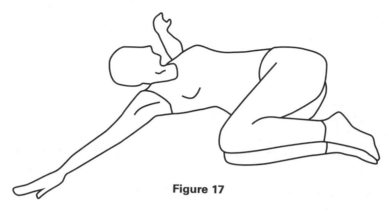

Figure 17

PRAYER
I am teachable.
Teach me what I need to know.
I surrender to your wisdom.
Aum.

Feel how relaxed your body is. Feel how peaceful you are as you surrender deeper and deeper into your own divinity.

Reverse sides now, moving your knees to the left and your head to the right. Keep the shoulders on the mat (fig. 18).

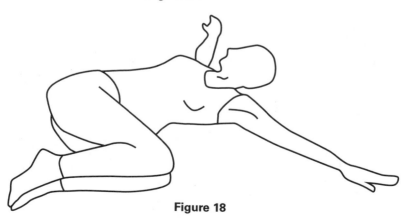

Figure 18

PRAYER
I surrender to you. Lead me home.
Lead me, beloved God of my being,
and I shall follow you.
I am yours now and forever.
Teach me. I am teachable.
Aum.

Return the legs back to center, extending and resting them. Feel the beauty of God within each cell, blessing you and loving you.

Gently and tenderly place your hands on your body, wherever they are drawn. Surrender into the healing energy flowing within you. As you continue to lie basking and bathing in God's love, say a prayer of thanksgiving.

PRAYER
Beloved God,
I give thanks for this moment of now.
I am in oneness with you,
serving you
and living you through me.
Amen, amen, and amen.

CHAPTER **11**

Purification of the Soul:
the Second Stage of Surrender

The second stage of surrender is a movement of the purification of the soul. You have created union with the divine within you through the first series of devotional surrender postures and prayers. The stronger this union grows, the faster you will transform the illusions and begin to embody the living light of truth. In this series, you discard anything you are ready to release using the yoga of surrender, sahaja yoga. You will also utilize hatha yoga as your body spontaneously and gracefully moves into the surrender posture. You have tapped into the infinite wisdom of the body, and it will automatically move your body into a surrender asana and begin to breathe through you the appropriate breath. This is pranayama yoga at its highest and clearest. As you practice the second stage of surrender, any blockage (or karma) is cleared in the practice of karma yoga. Because you have cleared the blockage, you are open and receptive to experiencing tantra and kundalini at a deeper and richer level. Power is added to the surrender through the prayer and spoken words of laya yoga.

The soul is a recorder of your experiences. It records what you have embraced emotionally to be used as a reference. When you have an experience, your soul searches itself for a similar memory that may have been an experience of love, abandonment, or betrayal. The body recalls feeling the sensation before. You may find yourself reacting to the circumstances of your life from your soul memory. When you react, you are out of control and at the effect of life.

Jesus says that the mind of the body holds the past. The mind of the body is our human appetite for instant gratification and our need for possession on the material plane. Because of past wounds, the mind of the body desires love, thinking that this will instantly gratify or fill the hole inside. When you surrender the wounds one by one, they transform and dissolve, and you are receptive to pure love. Then you have what you wanted, and the need no longer exists, freeing you from the past.

How the Soul Is Imprinted

Thought is lowered into emotion. Emotion is then lowered into matter. Once the body feels the impulse of the sensation of emotion, it is recorded into the soul, creating memory. Therefore, what we choose to think and feel is very important, because that is what we become at the cellular level. During each session of Sacred Heart Yoga, you engage your mind, body, emotions, and soul. You become a higher vibration cellularly, and your soul becomes educated and purified.

The soul goes with you into each lifetime. The soul is you. It brings with you the wisdom you have gained, along with the distorted consciousness (all that needs to heal) so that your soul can become educated and evolve.

You enter your soul when you begin to feel. Your passport into your spirit is emotion — deeply felt emotions of love and pain. That is why you are asked in the first stage of surrender to continuously feel the prayers and to feel your love for God. Remember, deep in the soul are the songs of love you wish to sing to God. In the second stage of surrender, you are asked to surrender into the pain so that you can be purified. In this stage of surrender, you experience movement of the soul and an opportunity for a miracle.

> ### TEACHING FROM JESUS
> In the state of surrender, the possibility for all things is available.

In this stage of surrender, the cells are cleansed, and they release the old structure of energy they have been holding, such as sadness, suffering, separation, pain, fear, and anger. Once this old structure dissipates, a new energy and new life can take its place.

Release the Need to Control

The state of surrender is an experience of building your faith and trust in God, the source of your good. It is also an experience of your vulnerability, your courage, and your strength. You are given the opportunity to surrender all that you are not. You are not your anger, your sadness, your illness, or the circumstances in your life. You are the truth of God, which is the goodness and grace of God's love and life.

You can decide what and how much you wish to surrender. You may choose to surrender a little bit or all of yourself and your situation. Through this process, a freedom awaits you. In order to get to the other side of your blockage, into the unknown state of freedom, you must be willing to be out of control in the moment of surrender. As the old consciousness is dissolved within, you will find your true God self. You will find that your truth and wisdom are within and always have been.

When you have a need — to be loved, accepted, or appreciated — then you will try to control others. Jesus says, "When you surrender your needs, you let go of control. Then you become the almighty, indwelling God, and you are free. Surrender the need to control. Your personality self is filled with the need to attain material possessions. You are driven to be perfect, accepted, smart, loved, beautiful, and successful. You try to control life to attain and fulfill these needs. It is an impossible task. You can only find true love and fulfillment through God. You are in control when you become one force, one focus, one with the Infinite Mind of God."

This wisdom will serve you to free yourself from your attachments and become adaptable. When you find yourself affected by other people's actions, immediately look inside to your need; then surrender it to be at peace once again.

In this state, you truly begin to look inside yourself, seeing your fears and needs. It takes courage to face your darkness, no longer running away from yourself and your good. Jesus says, "This is a vulnerable state, for in the moment of surrender, you have given up control. You must be out of control to gain true control of your life. This state of surrender, therefore, is an act of courage and strength."

The key to your development is to be willing to surrender into your darkness. Feel the pain that has been locked within you. This not only takes courage but also a profound desire to heal and be free. In the moment of true surrender, you give it to God. Speak aloud to give a voice to the darkness and the pain. This is crucial to the process of surrender. Your unhealed self must speak the words of surrender. Ask God to lift the darkness and pain from your heart, mind, body, and soul. God will take you by the hand and lead you into a new life.

When you surrender, you may experience the energy moving your head back. The Shakti, or Holy Spirit, may be so powerful that your body may arch or spontaneously go into its own movement, or asana. You may even find yourself bouncing inches off the mat. This energy is dissolving the old structure within you, allowing you to be open and receptive to the wisdom and the truth. As you develop your relationship with the God within through devotion, the Father/Mother becomes alive within you and responds to your prayers to be cleansed of your old energy patterns.

The first series of Sacred Heart Yoga movements and attunements set the stage for the transformational experience of this second series.

Preparation Exercises

This state of surrender is more than a word. It is an experience that must come from deep inside of your being. You must be ready to surrender your old ways and willing to give them to God so that they may be lifted. Please take the time to reflect and meditate on the exercises that follow. They will help prepare you for surrender.

When I go inside myself, I see a door. I am on one side in the darkness of my limited mind, living an illusion of unworthiness. On the other side of the door is the light of my freedom, and I hold the key that unlocks the door. The key is surrender. All I have to do is have the courage to surrender and walk through to the light.

Jesus would tell me, "I will show you the way Home to the beloved Father, but you, my beloved one, must do the unfolding. No one can do this for you. Each must do his or her own unfolding to enter into the kingdom of God's wealth. Feel your sadness, your fear, and your anger so that they may be transformed into joy. Worship God by the life that you live. Focus on your unfoldment, staying steadfast to the vision of God I Am, Christ I Am. Become the ideal of God, a Christ."

In this exercise, close your eyes and be with this message from Jesus. After a moment, answer the questions that follow.

What does this message mean to you?

_____

_____

_____

Do you allow yourself to feel your darkness? If yes, briefly describe a recent experience.

_____

_____

_____

How do you worship God by the life that you live?

_____

_____

How do you stay focused on your own unfoldment?

_____

_____

_____

> ### *TEACHING FROM JESUS*
> This is a vulnerable state, for in the moment of surrender, you have given up control. You must be out of control to gain true control of your life.

This state of surrender, therefore, is an act of courage and strength. In the next exercise, take a moment to contemplate this truth. Be with it, and let it resonate with your being. Look inside of yourself, asking the questions that follow. Then write what you realize about yourself in relation to this truth.

What part of you is ready to heal?

_____

_____

_____

What need are you ready to surrender?

_____

_____

_____

Are you willing to be out of control so that you can gain true control of this part of you?

_____

_____

_____

The Experience of Awakening the Spiritual Senses

The deeper you go into the darkness, the greater your rewards will be. As you open up to vulnerability — exposing your shame, guilt, sadness, hate, and anger to the God within and surrendering them — your darkness will be dissolved by the light and the love of God. Transformation occurs at the cellular level, and your soul is purified. Then you begin to awaken the spiritual senses that are within you. You will become more as God is, knowing what you need to know, feeling the love of God caress your cells, and hearing the words of love from the love and light within. The love will speak gentle, soft, and loving words of truth to you, and you will feel this energetically as love caressing you. The light speaks to you of the truth of God. Wisdom is brought to you, and you experience this wisdom energetically in your cells.

God is revealing to you the truth and imprinting it into your cells. As the imprinting continues, you become this wisdom and love cellularly, and it is alive and living in this dimension to be shared and experienced. Jesus would tell me, "It is time now to surrender and move into the light of God where all that you desire exists."

You must have trust that the unknown state of freedom will be there for you. And you must be willing to surrender your suffering, pain, or lack in order to experience this new life of freedom. You are your own jailer, keeping yourself locked in your illusion of unworthiness. Remember, you have the key to freedom, and it is surrender.

This movement of surrendering your darkness cannot be forced. Once you choose to begin the process of surrendering, you will unfold naturally. The darkness will begin to come to light piece by piece. This darkness must be ready to return home to the Father's house. Be patient with yourself, and have faith that you are moving into the light and love of God's kingdom. If you weren't moving, you wouldn't recognize this wisdom.

Surrender Prayer Exercise

In the next exercise, reach deep inside you, and write your own prayers of surrender. The wounded self must speak the words of surrender. Let your emotions come to the surface, being in the state of vulnerability. Remember, the prayers in the book are a guide. They were my prayers in the moment of writing. For personal results and transformation, you must surrender your wounds, saying this in the words of pain or anger that is bound up within you.

Free yourself by speaking the truth of your life experiences to the Mother within you. She is waiting to love you unconditionally and transform your past, freeing you to live in the joy of the moment with a future filled with all possibilities. Use the following keys to assist you:

- Be humble and vulnerable.
- Be willing.
- Have courage.

- Call on your strength.
- Make the choice.
- Trust God.

_____
_____
_____
_____
_____
_____
_____
_____
_____
_____
_____
_____
_____
_____
_____
_____
_____
_____
_____
_____
_____
_____

The Second Series of Surrender Postures

Let us work with the concept of self-judgment. Is your self-judge ready to be healed? Are you ready to choose to love yourself? If so, then accept your critical self, and surrender into this energy of self-judgment. Deeply feel this part of you, and when you're ready, let your self-judge surrender to God.

Lie on your back. Place your hands under your sit bones, palms down. This is the natural state of surrender that your body will move into as you surrender and activate your Shakti. Now let the energy take you up on your forearms (fig. 19). Arch your back, lifting the chest, and rest the top of your head on the mat.

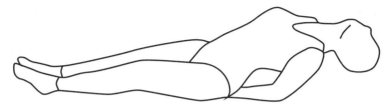

Figure 19.

PRAYER
Beloved indwelling Mother,
I willingly allow the structure of my critical self to dissipate.
I surrender my critical mind, my critical eye, my self-judgment,
and my self-hate so that I may love myself as I am.
Aum.

While in a sitting position, bend the right leg at the knee, and let the right foot come up on the outside of the leg. Keep the left leg straight, extended. Now, if you can, lie flat on your back and extend the arms above your head (fig. 20). You may also rest on the elbows, forearms, and hands if you are unable to lie down on your back (see fig. 22 for an alternate arm resting position). If you have knee limitations, you may not be comfortable in this position. Remember to always work at your own level of comfort.

As you speak the words of surrender, feel them deeply within your soul. When you speak from memories of a painful past, the soul is cleansed and purified.

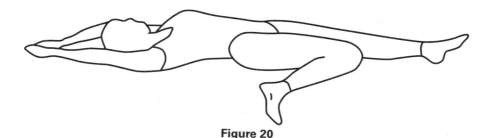

Figure 20

PRAYER
Beloved indwelling Mother,
I surrender whatever blockage I hold within my being
that keeps me separate from love — your love
and the love of those around me. And so it is.
Aum.

Come out of the posture, and resume a sitting position. Bend the left leg at the knee, and let the left foot come up on the outside of the leg. Keep your right leg straight, extended. Now, if you can, lie flat on your back and extend your arms above your head (fig. 21). Similar to the previous position, see fig. 22 for an alternate arm resting position if the position feels uncomfortable.

Now, with your mind, go into any part of yourself that holds back in matters of love, whether it's freely given or freely received. Let this part of you speak the prayer.

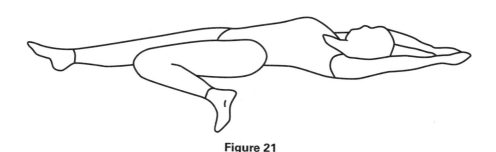

Figure 21

PRAYER
I open my heart to you, beloved Mother.
Cleanse me of this old fear. Heal me, heal me, and heal me.

I am yours. I desire to know of love fully and completely.

Heal me so that I may live in the river of love with no fear, no hate,

no separation — only love, joy, and abundance.

Hear my prayer, beloved Mother.

Hear my prayer. And so it is.

Aum.

From a seated position, bend both knees, and bring your feet outside the legs. Stay in this seated position, and place your hands on the mat next to your hips, fingers pointing away from the body. If you are able, go back down onto your elbows and forearms (fig. 22).

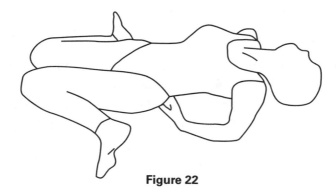

Figure 22

If you can, lie flat on your back and extend your arms above your head (fig. 23).

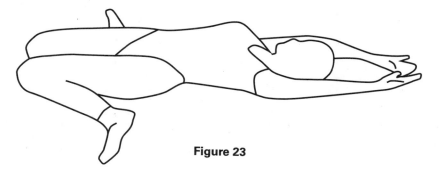

Figure 23

PRAYER

Beloved Mother,

I surrender to you this fear of being loved completely
and of loving completely.

Take this fear from my mind, my body, my heart, and my soul
so that I may serve you more fully.

Aum.

CHAPTER 12

The Law of Acceptance

Once you have gone through the stages of surrender, you enter the second stage of Sacred Heart Yoga in which you will apply the law of acceptance. Accept the truth, for the truth shall set you free.

Acceptance Begins the Healing Process

As you accept the truth, whether it is the false truth you have held about yourself or the actual truth of God, your first seal and chakra will begin to expand. When you accept a false concept, your first sacred seal opens a pathway to the heart, and in that moment, healing begins. You have left the state of denial. Because this is the seal and chakra of your life force energy, you will instantly have more life energy flowing through your body.

When you accept a false truth about yourself, such as thinking, "I am afraid I'll do something wrong," you instantly leave the state of denial. When you live in the state of denial, you are truly dying. To enter the state of living and generating new life energy in the first sacred seal, all you need to do is accept your feelings and limited beliefs about yourself and life.

Once you truly become truthful with yourself and begin the process of accepting your darkness, this new life energy that you have created within you moves up the central nervous system to the brain. The brain then begins to awaken from its dead sleep. You then are free to accept the truth about yourself, and a new energy will be sent throughout your system to every cell in the body. You are regenerating your physical, emotional, and mental bodies with God's truth.

Each time you move from the darkness of your own beliefs to accepting the truth, you string a pearl of wisdom on the silver thread of eternal life. When your silver thread is filled with your own jewels of wisdom, you will be illuminated. All of your blockages will be dissolved by the light of truth, the light of God.

There are two phases of acceptance. The first deals with identifying and accepting the incorrect concepts and the false truths you hold about yourself and life. The second phase deals with accepting the correct concepts and the new truth about yourself and life.

The First Phase of Acceptance

If at any time in the past, you accepted that you are not good enough to receive or have what you truly want, then that energy is locked within you. This outdated energy keeps you from your dreams and the power to manifest them.

> ### TEACHING FROM JESUS
> Your limited thoughts destroy you and cause you to age, suffer, and live in pain. You die because you don't realize the truth.

If you lack in anything — love, money, or health — then look inside, and examine the hidden concepts you emanate to the world that say you are not worthy or good enough. Begin to move into surrendering them to God.

Often, children are told that they are good or the opposite, that they are bad, and then they believe it. Jesus says, "It is done unto you as you believe." If you think you are good, the world will treat you as if you are good, giving you love, acceptance, and appreciation. The world merely validates your truth. The reverse is also true: To the degree you have embraced that you are bad, you will be treated badly. You will be ignored, criticized, forgotten, and so on. The world says, "You think you are unworthy, so I will treat you accordingly." You then blame those who mistreat you and take on the role of a victim.

When you take responsibility for what you have conceived about yourself, you then have the power to change. As soon as you accept the false truth that you have conceived, it will begin to dissipate. When you become honest with yourself, seeing and feeling your pain, it frees you instantly. But often, we hide from ourselves and pretend that everything is fine. We run away from ourselves by keeping busy or becoming workaholics, or we cover our pain with sex, alcohol, drugs, sugar, shopping, caffeine, cigarettes, or any other addictive form that alters our pain. These are all forms of self-abuse and self-hate.

When Jesus was teaching me, he would stop me in one of these behaviors, interrupting me in the middle of my pattern, saying, "Face yourself. Once you face your false truth or fearful self, it will lose power over you." He would tell me that this false truth (the fearful self or self-hatred) was my devil, or evil self, and that I could dissolve it by just standing still and facing it head on. It took a tremendous amount of courage, but I did just that and found that it works. It is very scary in the beginning, but it helps to know that you're not alone. God is always with you to support you through your darkness into the light.

Jesus also explained that when I held an incorrect concept and truly believed it, that this was a false god I had put before me. So when you begin to accept the truth, you are loving, honoring, and worshipping God.

TEACHING FROM JESUS
You worship God by the life you live.

When you take responsibility for what you think about yourself, you then have the power to change, to be free from the incorrect concepts and false beliefs. You must first begin to empty out the old concepts and beliefs before you can begin to imprint the new concept.

There are two steps to dissolving the darkness of false truths and incorrect concepts:

1. By accepting yourself exactly as you are, you are set free. If you are afraid, you must accept that you are afraid. Whatever it is, accept it. This starts the flow of energy that begins to dissolve the blockages. Say a prayer of acceptance for your fear.

   PRAYER
   Beloved God, I accept that I'm afraid
   there isn't enough for me and that this isn't the truth.

   Be specific, and talk to God as a dear friend who truly loves and cares for you. Tell God everything with honesty and vulnerability, and don't hold anything back.

2. Face the fearful self, and surrender the fear and pain to God. Through surrender, the incorrect concept begins to be lifted and erased from your soul memory, and then you are free to create whatever truth you choose. You can proceed with accepting the new truth, embracing the new truth, and becoming this new truth. The following is an example of surrendering through prayer.

PRAYER

Beloved God, I surrender my fear that there isn't enough for me.
I give this to you. Take it. Take it from my body,
from my heart, from my soul, and from my mind.
Thank you, beloved God. I no longer need this fear.
It is not the truth, and I am ready to let it go and live the truth.

The Second Phase of Acceptance

By accepting the truth of God, you will quicken the vibrations of the body, allowing you to begin vibrating the frequencies of truth. This cleanses your aura, stills your mind, and purifies your soul. You will begin to embody the truth of God, and this truth will be transmitted back to the mind of God and the river of consciousness. These higher frequencies will assist in purifying the planet. When the truth of God is embodied within your flesh, you will live the truth for others to see. It is no longer only available in higher realms of consciousness but also living in the world. The truth of God will emanate from within you.

Jesus says, "Accept the thoughts of truth. Use your thoughts of love, peace, and harmony to build the mansion within. As you accept the truth by experiencing the oneness, then the truth will become knowledge, and it will be imprinted into your consciousness, your cells, and your soul. Then you will vibrate this wisdom forever. You will become the love of God. The Father within you will become you, expressing freely through you."

Acceptance is the first step in manifestation. Change in your inner world will then be reflected in your outer world.

There are five steps to vibratory transformation:

1. Accept the truth, the new concept you have about yourself or your life.
2. Embrace the truth, feeling the new concept. It is through feeling the new truth that it becomes you. It is recorded into the soul and imprinted into every cell of your human body. Whatever you become will be your outer world experience.
3. Know the truth, the new concept of self or life. Through the embracing process, the new concept becomes knowledge within you because it is you. You must feel something to know it. Then you will know who you are.
4. Experience the truth, the new concept of self or life. You will have experiences that validate this in your life because you will magnetically draw similar vibrations to you. The world is a reflection of who you are and what you feel and know about yourself.

5. Be the truth, the new concept. Being is the result of accepting and embracing a concept of truth. You experience being the concept you have embraced.

The world reflects back to you your new concept, creating the experience of a new life.

Become What You Want to Manifest or Experience in Life

You will find your world becoming different, and you will attract new friends, a new life, and new experiences to mirror your new truth. This is the process of creating a new world. The power is within you to create whatever you need to fulfill your soul. I love sharing this because it works easily and rapidly. It is so exciting. All you need is the courage and strength to dive into the pain of the old concepts and surrender them to God.

This process of transformation in Sacred Heart Yoga is very complete. In other forms of therapy, you empty out by feeling fear, rage, sadness, or other difficult feelings, but they don't transform completely. In the Sacred Heart Yoga experience of transformation, you work with the science of the body, and then you work with God as your partner or therapist. God has the power to erase the old frequencies of thought that created the imbalance.

It is essential to fill the void with a new imprint, a new vibration. That is why you accept the new truth, embracing it so that you can become the truth of God. Your soul is then educated, and your body becomes obedient to your spirit. You will express the higher vibrations of God through you.

TEACHING FROM JESUS
Holding the Truth

When you hold the truth of yourself in consciousness, you can only experience yourself as divine. You can never change anything. You can rise above disease and disharmony to the spiritual truth, and the disease or disharmony will then begin to dissolve and change form. So do not deny your fears; face them, and move your consciousness to the spiritual plane, the one mind of God, where all truth is available and waiting to be accessed and lived. Humankind grows by realizing the truth of itself, expanding consciousness, and opening to the God within, to the truth that is waiting to be lived in each moment.

This wisdom from Jesus took me a long time to truly understand. You can never change anything. You can rise to the spiritual truth that is above disease and disharmony, making them dissolve and change form.

Now I understand that my old concepts are my illusions, and what I experience in my life is what I have embraced as the truth. It is my ego that embraced those concepts. The ego always wants to be right and in control. It wants to manipulate and change through force. This doesn't work, as I'm sure you have experienced. Now when I see and accept my darkness, or incorrect concept, I can surrender it to God. As God lifts it, I can embrace the spiritual truth. That is how I can dissolve the disharmony or disease and rise above it to the truth to experience a new life of harmony, ease, and joy.

CHAPTER 13

The I Am Principle

The I Am principle is a formula for changing the totality of your being at the cellular level. You work directly with the soul in this series of asanas and prayers. The soul records what you feel. As you embrace the prayers of truth that you speak, you transform from density into light.

You will use hatha yoga and laya yoga in the series of I Am postures and prayers. Spontaneous breathing — pranayama yoga — may also begin as your vibration quickens. Pranayama is the breath of life that dwells within you. As you practice the series of I Am prayers and postures, the flow of your creative energy and the flow of your passion energy will weave and intermingle to begin the dance of tantra yoga within you. Your sacred energy will then begin to carouse up through your spine and central nervous system, activating your kundalini. This is kundalini yoga.

The key to the development of this series is to feel the new concepts as you speak the words of wisdom and truth. Feel and embrace your words as fully and completely as you can. You must become your feelings and thoughts. They must become you. Bring the feelings from deep within your soul so that they can spring forth into life.

This series of asanas brings balance and harmony to the male and female in your entire being. It creates a marriage, a union between the male and female energies in each cell of your body. A cellular renewal and reunion will also occur within each cell.

The *I* in the I Am is male, and the *Am* in the I Am is female. The purpose and the function of the female is to feel and embrace. The female becomes whatever she embraces and is creation. She creates by conceiving concepts and by feeling them. When you hold a concept of life, or of self, and embrace it, you conceive this concept into your total being, body and soul.

TEACHING FROM JESUS

If person is to bring forth the Holy Spirit through him- or herself, he or she must embrace all that God is.

This means that you must be willing to surrender limited self-perceptions. The truth of God certainly isn't our deep, dark feelings of self. In healing myself and others for many years, I have found that we don't like ourselves very much. Many of us feel less than godly and godlike.

You must begin to allow the ego to transform into its true godliness. The ego must become humble and be pure in its desire to become as God is. This returns us to our original state. You already are all you could ever want to be, but you forget and put layer on layer of false concepts over the true beauty of God that you are.

When the *Am* embraces that it is godlike and godly, then the *I* becomes these qualities that have been embraced and expresses them into life. The male has the function of broadcasting the concept conceived to every cell of the body as a messenger of your perceptions of life. He then sends this frequency out into your energy field, telling the world around you what you have conceived. The world then responds to you according to your vibration. You magnetize to you a like vibration, and you have an experience that validates your truth. This is the mirror process; that is, we are what we see in others.

As an example, if you embrace the concept that you are love, you begin to become the identity of love and express love into life. God has many qualities, and as you embrace each one, you become that quality and have a new identity. Your true identity becomes available to live through you, and it is no longer distorted by the false perceptions of self. If in the past your identity was to think that you are less than godly, then that is what you expressed. It was the image of self you lived. Is it any wonder that things didn't work out smoothly?

The I Am principle is an embodying experience. We have all held a tremendous amount of information in our intellect that we could spout out to look great. There is a problem with this: It doesn't belong to us. We don't own it. It's just lip service because it hasn't become who we are. We then can't walk our talk.

As you embody the truth, the God within you expresses through you in the way you walk, talk, and move through life because that God truth is you. The same is true when you have embodied a God quality. You feel the energy of the God quality moving through you. When you have embodied love, love moves through you, and it feels blissful. If you have embodied power and certainty, you feel secure in yourself as these energies move through you. Feeling the God qualities that you have embodied moving in and through you is indescribably delicious.

When you begin to embody a new truth, you become the electrical vibration of that new truth. The *Am* (the negative energy) embraces the new concept of God, and that electrical frequency is sent from cell to cell by the *I* (the positive energy). As this occurs, your body will experience a quickening within as your vibration becomes faster and higher. Your limbs may even begin to move uncontrollably, as in kriya.

I see this as one cell tapping the cell next to it, broadcasting the good news from cell to cell throughout the entire body — a chain reaction moving throughout the cellular structure. If I embrace love, the cells would begin to share the news: "I am love. I am love. I am love," from cell to cell, until my entire body vibrates at the frequency of love. Then I would have become love in physical form. My spirit, which is love, would be alive in each cell expressing freely into life through my eyes, smile, walk, talk, and actions. That brings forth the Holy Spirit through me into life.

The *I* is to realize and to live as an individual expression of God. Then the *I* expresses through uniqueness and perfection, no longer striving to conform and be like others. This energy no longer tries to be better than others because the *I* knows that he is a perfect, pure, and beautiful expression of God, living through a human body. He appreciates his gifts, realizing that there is no one exactly like him.

The I Am Series of Postures

Always begin on the left side with these arm postures. The left side is the feminine, or the Am, side of the body. From your lying-down position, raise the left arm straight up to the heavens. Slowly let the energy move your arm across the body to the right. Place the right hand between the shoulder and elbow joints and gently press downward to assist you in extending the stretch and opening the shoulder (fig. 24).

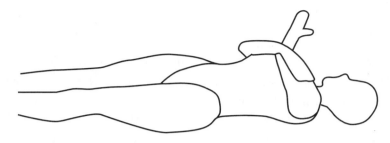

Figure 24

Close your eyes, and embrace the words of the prayer.

PRAYER
I choose to accept that God's goodness is within me.
I choose to accept that God's grace moves through me.
I choose to accept that I am one and the same as God's goodness.
I choose to accept that I am one and the same as God's grace.
Aum.

Release your left arm, returning it to the mat. Feel the energy of goodness and grace that you are creating.

Raise the right arm straight up to the heavens. Slowly let the energy move the arm across your body to the left as far as it will go. Place the hand between the shoulder and elbow joints, and gently press downward to assist you in extending the stretch and opening the shoulder (fig. 25).

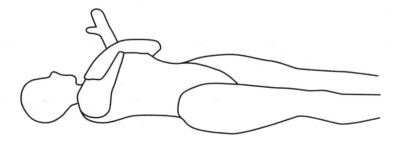

Figure 25

PRAYER
I can accept God's goodness is within me.
I can accept God's grace moves through me.
I can accept that I am one and the same
as God's goodness and grace.
I can express goodness and grace into life.
Aum.

Release the right arm, and feel the energy transmitting this truth into life.
Place the left arm out from the shoulder, palm facing down. Bring the right
hand over your left ear, and guide the head to the right (fig. 26). Gently open and
stretch the left side of your neck and shoulder.

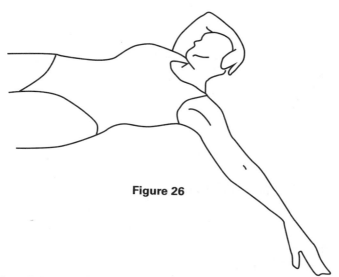

Figure 26

As you embrace that the abundance of God's wealth is within you, God's abundance will become more available to you.

PRAYER
I choose to embrace abundance.
I choose to accept that there is enough abundance for me.
I choose to embody the abundance of God's wealth.
Aum.

Release the right hand, and let the head return to center. Feel the energy moving all around you in your electromagnetic field.

Place the right arm straight out from your shoulder, palm facing down. Bring the left hand over the right ear, and guide the head to the left (fig. 27). Gently open and stretch the right side of the neck and right shoulder.

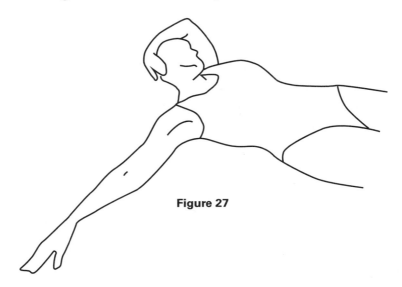

Figure 27

The male *I* brings you whatever you have embraced. If you have embraced abundance, then this abundance is brought to you from all sources, both from within and also from the world around you.

PRAYER
I can accept that there is enough for me.
I can embrace abundance.
I can live abundantly.
Aum.

Release the left hand, and let the head return to center. Feel the atmosphere that is around you. Your consciousness has been raised, and the energy has quickened. You are transmitting a new frequency into the universe.

The Temple

The temple series is from ancient Egypt and includes the divine dance of tantra, kundalini, hatha, laya, sahaja, bhakti, and beloved raja yoga practices. While in the mummy asana, you will dive deeply into a blissful state of raja yoga. Your brain waves will change, taking you easily into raja, a deep state of meditation.

The temple is a series of four asanas and mudras: the tabernacle, the temple of eternal life, the temple flow, and the mummy. These temple movements are very powerful and very pleasurable to your entire being. They are asanas and mudras of energy, pure divine energy.

Without conscious thought, the energy will move your hands in an ancient mudra flow that was taught in the Egyptian mystery schools. You already know these movements, as your soul remembers them. These movements take you into the DNA system of the body, the system of wisdom, knowledge, and creation. Your body will create geometric symbols throughout this temple series.

You will connect the male and female energies, and the body will begin a movement of giving and receiving from within. The energy flows between the male and female in a figure eight (the symbol of infinity). You may feel a rocking motion as you progress in these movements. The rib cage will begin to move back and forth as the male and female energies intertwine and dance together. It is a very sensual yet peaceful feeling. Your male and female energies come into balance. As you develop these energies within, your bones begin to float and align themselves.

You must surrender to the intelligence of the divine energy and rely on it, allowing the energy to have full sway in your body. Let it manifest within you. Give it permission to finally move in and through you.

The Tabernacle

The tabernacle is created over the heart sacred seal and chakra. Within the tabernacle is the chalice, or Holy Grail, that is filled with the kingdom of God, God's wealth, everything we could ever want or need. Clairvoyants in my classes have described the chalice as jeweled and incredibly beautiful.

In this asana, you take whatever you need or want, and you drink freely from the chalice, letting it fill you. If you find a lack or emptiness within, you drink from the chalice, allowing it to fill every need, every lack in your life. It is not only symbolic — it uses the mind and the senses to experience being filled from within — but also energetic: You become the energy of whatever you drink from the chalice.

For example, if you feel lonely, then drink of love and companionship, and the energy of loneliness will dissolve and be filled with love. You will then manifest companionship and love in your life.

The key to activating the flow of God's wealth is to realize that the kingdom of God is within you. As you realize that and drink of your own wealth, the chalice begins to overflow with joy.

The purpose of drinking from the chalice is to be filled from within, to receive whatever you need in the moment from the kingdom of God's wealth within. As you practice this posture, you discover and begin to activate the divinity within you.

The Tabernacle Posture

Lie down, placing the soles of your feet together. Bring the palms of your hands together over the heart in prayer mudra. Allow yourself to feel the balancing within the body. Feel the peace of this positive-negative flow of energy as you give and receive within yourself. Let the energy move your hands up over the heart seal and chakra, stopping halfway up (fig. 28).

Enter the tabernacle with the mind and senses. You find within a beautiful chalice. The Holy Grail is within you. In this chalice lies everything you need. Rejoice in this knowledge. Everything is within your heart.

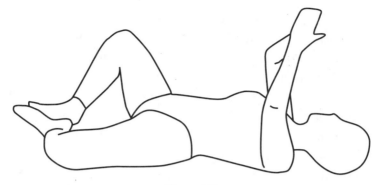

Figure 28

PRAYER
I drink of love.
I drink of perfect health.
I drink of peace and joy.
I drink of abundance.
Aum.

Drink freely of everything you want and need. Feel the energy filling you and freely flowing through you.

PRAYER
I give myself what I have longed for
and have never received from others.
I realize that everything
is within me, and I am filled.
I give myself All That God Is
that I Am.
I am safe in my body,
and I am safe in my life,
for I Am as God Is,
and there is nothing I need.
Aum.

Lie in peace. Peace, be still. The body needs to be in peace to heal.

The Temple of Eternal Life Posture

This asana signifies that the body is filled with the life of God. It is an opportunity to love your body, seeing it as God created it, perfect and divine. Once you begin to love your body, the body can begin to become the vibration of love. Healing can then occur instantly. You begin to regenerate new cells with the vibration of love and acceptance of self.

Let the hands move up over your head. This creates a pyramid over the crown of the head. Your legs remain in a pyramid form under the root seal (fig. 29). The two double pyramids you are forming create a tremendous amount of power. Symbols are a way of creating energy and can also be used as doorways into other dimensions and into the DNA.

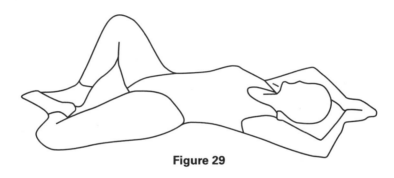

Figure 29

PRAYER
I love you, body.
You are beautiful, body.
You are the life of God, body, and I love you.
Aum.

You may feel it appropriate to forgive yourself for expecting the body to be something God didn't create it to be or for judging the body through your expectations to look a certain way.

PRAYER OF FORGIVENESS
I forgive myself for not accepting my body,
for not loving my body.
I forgive myself for judging my body
and expecting it to be something

to please the consciousness of the material world.
Aum.

Repeat a prayer of love for your body.

PRAYER
I love you, body.
You are beautiful exactly as you are.
Body, you were created to express love
through your eyes, your voice,
your movements,
and your touch.
Aum.

The Temple Flow Postures

The temple flow is designed to acknowledge the light within the body. This mudra movement will create a divine flow of energy. You repeat this movement three times.

The purpose of this movement is to dive into the darkness and bring light and wisdom to the unhealed self, bringing the divine energy into human form. There is a natural flow of energy that moves from the crown to the root seal in a loop. When you are disconnected from the truth, this flow of energy is interrupted, making you feel out of balance. You are reconnecting the divine flow within you. This movement is a soul retrieval, which frees you from your limited illusions of self and life. You acknowledge yourself by anointing yourself. When you touch your lips, you are blessing yourself. You bring this energy of anointing and blessing into the heart.

From the heart, turn your hands downward, pointing toward the root seal, where you dive into the lower aspects of consciousness and energy to the personality self, unhealed self or ego. Then bring your hands back from the root to the crown over your head, sounding the Aum. This cleanses and dissolves the old, limited energy as it ascends from the lower seals and chakras into the light.

It is a great act of love and compassion for self. You are finally beginning to love your darkness. Healing occurs when you have love and compassion for yourself.

The First Flow

Let the hands move over the forehead (fig. 30).

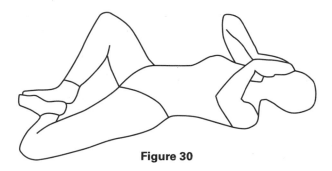

Figure 30

PRAYER
I anoint myself,
all that lives within my body.
I anoint my fears and my strengths.
Aum.

Let the hands move down to your lips, kissing your thumbs as they pass over the lips.

PRAYER
I bless all that I am.
I bless my fears and my strengths.
Aum.

Now let the energy move your hands to the heart center (fig. 31).

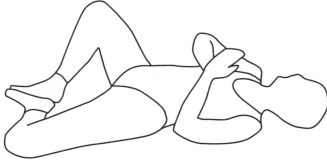

Figure 31

Turn the hands downward, and allow them to move down to the root seal (fig. 32).

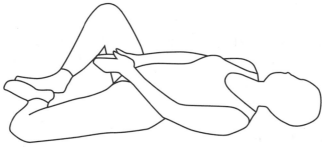

Figure 32

PRAYER
I dive into my human self, and I bring myself compassion,
understanding, and love.
I bring tenderness to myself.
I praise myself for my willingness to be here,
to look at myself and be honest.
And I ascend my doubts now.
Aum.

Bring your hands from the root to the crown (fig. 33).

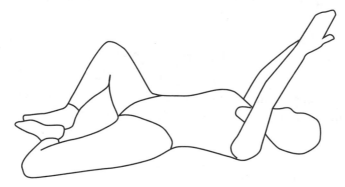

Figure 33

The Second Flow

Once again, allow the grace of God to move your hands. Gently touch the forehead repeating the hand position of figure 30.

PRAYER
I anoint my fearful self.

Allow the grace to move the hands down to your lips. As you pass over the lips, kiss your thumbs.

PRAYER
Blessed be I
who seeks the truth of God.

Bring your hands down to your heart (fig. 31), and point your hands downward, diving into your human self (fig. 32).

PRAYER
I dive into my unworthiness,
and I tell my unworthy self,
"You are worthy of God's love,
God's life, and God's kingdom."
I ascend my unworthiness.
Aum.

Sound the Aum, and return your hands from the root to the crown, above the head (fig. 33).

The Third Flow

You will move your hands from above your head (the crown) to the base of the spine (the root seal and chakra) and then return your hands back up to the crown to complete the third flow as in figures 30 through 33.

PRAYER
I anoint myself as God's perfect child,
perfect life, and perfect creation.

I bless the life that I Am.
I bless my humanness.

I dive into my guilt.
I bless my guilt and return it
to God's light and love
to be dissolved.
Aum.

I am holy,
I am sacred,
and I am beloved of God.
Aum.

Gently and slowly allow yourself to come out of this asana.

Any time your back is out of alignment or hurting, you can do this asana. Surrender to the intelligence of your divine energy.

Jane, a student of Sacred Heart Yoga, shares her experience of doing the temple flow: I've been doing this posture for a while, and I didn't have an explanation of this process. I have scoliosis, and it has been helping tremendously. Things in my back begin to snap, move, break loose, and correct. I found that I can move my hands over the seals and chakras, and different parts of my spine move.

The Mummy Posture

The purpose of the mummy asana is to create the state of infinite love of self. This asana seals you in your own love. When you cross the right ankle over the left, it blocks outside energy from entering your field and body. And when you cross your arms over the heart seal and center, the divine flow of love is sealed in. Your female gives love, tenderness, and compassion to the male as he gives strength, wisdom, power, and protection to her. In this asana, you feel relaxed and complete. You have come into balance with your male and female.

In the mummy, you will hold yourself in your own love and light, finding peace, fulfillment, and contentment within yourself. There is a meridian at the top of the arms where you place the hands that allows love to enter the heart seal and chakra from the male and female, or positive and negative, energy flows. This creates total balance within. The energy moves in a figure eight, the symbol of infinity. Infinite love of self is felt energetically, which leads to accepting the male, or doer, in us. It also leads to letting go of expectations of self and our feelings of failure. The female begins to appreciate all that the male is doing in life to provide for her. And the male, in turn, dedicates his life to loving, protecting, and providing for the female. She then can be the love that nourishes him.

Place the right ankle over the left. Cross your arms over the heart seal and center to form an X over the heart with the right arm over the left. Now place your left hand on your upper right arm just below the shoulder. Then place your right hand on your upper left arm just below the shoulder (fig. 34).

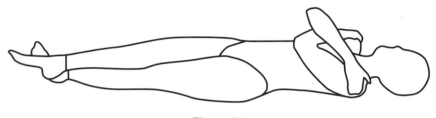

Figure 34

PRAYER
I protect myself,
for I am safe within myself —
safe to dwell within my
own love of self
and love of God.
Aum.

Rest in this posture for a few moments until you feel complete. Then slowly and gently release your hands and feet, and roll to your side, rolling into the fetal position. Finally, use your hands to assist you into a seated position.

15

The Principle of Desire and Will

The dance of the Goddess comes alive in this series of Sacred Heart Yoga asanas and prayers. You will use a combination of hatha, laya, bhakti, and pranayama yoga practices to begin effortlessly moving the energy throughout your system. The dance of the Goddess and the God will emerge from your solar plexus, and the tantra of Goddess/God will begin to weave love through you. Kundalini will truly be present as the Goddess comes alive and lives her dance within you.

Each of us has an inner female and inner male, even if we express through either a male or female embodiment. The purpose of the desire and will asana and prayer is to bring harmony and balance within our own male and female. The divinity of the third chakra resides in the sacred seal, which holds the Goddess-God. This divinity is developed as you practice the asana and prayers. The Goddess is the energy of desire, which is the aspect you will develop in this practice. Her function is to desire to serve God, to feel her love for the God within (her male counterpart) and the God in All That Is. She does this through yielding to her male counterpart, desiring to love him. And he, in turn, desires to serve her. He serves her through honoring her desires, which are her feelings and intuition, and through his deeds and actions. He also serves the Goddess within himself and the Goddess in All That Is in the same way.

In working with this asana, you will find that it is no longer your human will but Divine will that will lead you home into God's kingdom.

The energy that turns the key in this posture is desire. You must feel the essence and energy of pure desire. Desire is without need or desperation. It is not commanding or controlling. Through the process of feeling desire, you become the pure essence of the Goddess and her energy of desire.

In order to bring balance and harmony within, both the female and male must fulfill their functions. The function of the female is to lead the male home to God, desiring to serve God. The function of the male is to serve the female and to honor her feelings. The will fulfills the desires of the Goddess. Feelings ignite the life within you. The Goddess must feel her love if she is to ignite and manifest the life she has chosen. The Goddess and her desire is the spark behind the flame, and the flame is the will of God. She must be filled with a burning desire to ignite the flame; the stronger her desire, the greater his flame will be.

TEACHING FROM JESUS

The flesh is to be illuminated by the light that is ignited within (the female function) and birthed forth into life (male function). The male gives birth to the light through his actions and deeds.

As the third sacred seal is developed, the breath of manifestation will occur spontaneously. The energy of desire will be released from within the third seal, and it will move up the energy system and out the top of your head. The muscles in the solar plexus will contract, pumping the energy, while the breath spontaneously assists and moves the energy up and out. As this phenomenon occurs, you literally become the true essence of desire and will.

TEACHING FROM JESUS

Your desire and will must be in harmony, both in service to the unfoldment of the Christ in you.

This means that the Goddess in you must have a pure desire to know God, to serve God, to feel God, and to be one with God. God's will must be ready to serve the Goddess through his actions and deeds, honoring the Goddess and her desires.

In life, men who have powerful women behind them go forth to accomplish miracles, bringing bountiful fruit home to the Goddess. The female is to believe in and have faith in her male within and in the man in her life. Women, if you find doubt or weakness in your mate, the same weakness and doubt is within your inner male. If you judge or criticize your mate, you are judging and condemning your own male within. If you love him in his weakness and encourage, praise, and believe in him, he will grow to fulfill his destiny. The male is to serve the female, honoring and caring about her feelings and intuition. When the male is in service to the female, he is living according to his divine nature, and he is fulfilled. He truly wants to provide abundantly for her, protect her, care for her, and satisfy her sexually. He needs the love, approval, and encouragement of the female in order to serve her fully.

Honor is a quality of the knight. As the male grows and feels less threatened, he is able to honor the female because he is empowered by her. Men, if you are not honoring the feelings and intuition of the female in your life, you are not honoring the feminine within you. A male who honors his female within and the woman in his life honors himself.

Honor is born when you live your heart's desire. This creates dominion over your life. In the state of honor, there is no settling for less than what your heart desires.

Fulfill Your Desires

TEACHING FROM JESUS

Your prayers must be pure and honest, coming from your heart, coming from the sweetness of your soul. They must be filled with desire to be ful-filled. Dive deep into your soul, bringing your desires to the God within, the source of all of your good. Once you send forth your desire, let God (the male) bring it to you. The how, the when, and the where are left to God. It will come into form even greater than you could have imagined. Trust God to bring to you your desires, and let God do his work. Do not engage your ego mind. If fears and doubts begin to plague you, surrender them. Return to accepting and trusting the power of God (your male).

As you become desire and choose to serve God, the will of God springs forth from your soul and fulfills your desires through manifestation. This principle, when realized in relationships, creates harmony, joy, and an abundant shared life, and each person fulfills his or her function and purpose. The power struggle then ends in relationships between men and women.

TEACHING FROM JESUS

Putting God first — this is the right way to live, and it assures that your life will be fruitful and bountiful. All your needs will be provided for abun-dantly.

As you become desire, the old energy of control and dominance will be dissolved, and you will be free to create from within yourself peace and harmony between your own male and female selves. This will be mirrored in your male and female relationships in this human dimension.

Desire and Will Exercises

As children, many of us were criticized. When no one believed in us or encouraged us, our male energy became damaged. The female also became damaged if we were rejected for a part of our intuition or our love, joy, or innocence. As damaged and wounded ones, we didn't grow in godliness.

Now take a look at how desire and will have been working in your life by asking the child within (the wounded self) these questions, and write what you find.

Are you ready to feel your desire to know God?

_____

_____

_____

_____

_____

Is it your will to serve God?

_____

_____

_____

_____

If you found resistance in your child, go back to the first instance when you were wounded and begin to correct the error in consciousness. Begin to whisper the truth of God to the child. Continue to work with the child until he or she is ready to accept the truth.

Take a moment to look at your willingness in life by reflecting on these questions.

Are you willing to honor your feelings?

_____

_____

How?

_____

_____

The Goddess is the intuitive part of you. Are you willing to honor your desires and your intuition?

_____

_____

_____

_____

How?

_____

_____

In your relationship with your partner, do you choose to serve him or her?

_____

_____

Are you willing to honor this person's feelings and intuition?

_____

_____

_____

If you found resistance, find out why. Write down what you are resisting.

_____

_____

_____

_____

Now that you have found your belief or distorted perception, you can begin to correct it by whispering the truth to yourself. Jesus often whispered the truth to me in my morning meditations. For half an hour or more, he repeated one single truth over and over until I began to accept it and let it in. As I let the truth in, I usually cried as my wall of fear and old beliefs dissolved. Now I whisper and repeat over and over to myself whatever truth I need to embody so that I can change my consciousness and become that truth. This could take a day, a week, a month, or longer, depending on how large the blockage or how deep the wound is that needs healing.

Here is an example of whispering the truth to yourself. Suppose you find a belief that says, "You can't trust your intuition." Counter it by whispering to yourself, "You can trust your intuition. There's something within you that knows." Repeat it over and over until you begin to feel it inside. Jesus says that we have specific cells that make up the subconscious mind. As children, whatever we were told or perceived as true is what was recorded in the subconscious mind. The subconscious mind can be reprogrammed by repeating the truth over and over each day until the old programming is completely dissolved and a new program is in place.

The Desire and Will Posture

In the posture for the left side, begin with the right leg straight out in front of you. Bend the left knee, and bring the left leg over the right, planting the left foot on the mat just outside of the right knee. This signifies the female crossing over the male.

Bring the right arm around the left knee, pulling the knee toward your chest. Sit up straight and tall, lifting up out of the rib cage and elongating your spine. Raise your left arm, gazing at the left hand as you slowly bring this hand behind you, twisting the torso and shoulders. When you can go no further, bring the left hand down to the mat, and place it as close to the sacrum as possible (fig. 35).

As you breathe in, lift up out of the rib cage, elongating the spine, and as you breathe out, twist the torso to the left, keeping your sit bones on the mat. Repeat this several more times by breathing in and elongating the spine, then breathing out and twisting.

The breath of manifestation may spontaneously occur. You may begin to breathe very rapidly as the energy of desire is released from the third seal. This energy will move up and out the top of your head, cascading all around you.

If you are ready to come into harmony with your male-female within, then say the prayers, feeling the words as they spring forth from deep within your gut (solar plexus).

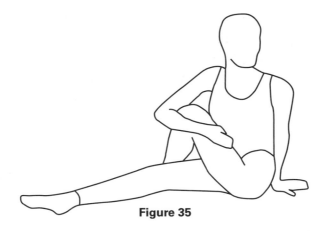

Figure 35

PRAYER
Desire I am. Desire I am.
Desire I am.
I desire to live for you,
my beloved God.
I desire to know you fully
and to serve you fully.
Aum.

In the posture for the right side, begin with the left leg straight out in front of you. Bend the right knee, and bring the right leg over the left, planting the right foot on the mat just outside of the left knee. This signifies the male crossing over the female.

Bring the left arm around the right knee, pulling the knee toward your chest. Sit up straight and tall, lifting up out of the rib cage and elongating your spine. Raise your right arm, gazing at the right hand as you slowly bring this hand behind you, twisting the torso and shoulders. When you can go no further, bring the right hand down to the mat, and place it as close to the sacrum as possible (fig. 36).

As you breathe in, lift up out of the rib cage, elongating the spine, and as you breathe out, twist the torso to the right, keeping your sit bones on the mat. Repeat this several more times by breathing in and elongating the spine, then breathing out and twisting.

The breath of manifestation may spontaneously occur. You may begin to breathe very rapidly as the energy of will is released from the third seal. This energy will move up and out the top of your head, cascading all around you. If you are ready to begin entering into harmony with your feelings and knowingness, then say the prayer from deep within you.

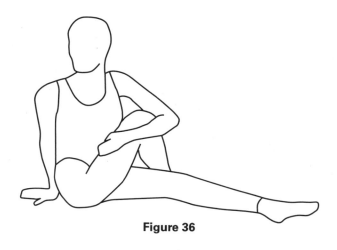

Figure 36

PRAYER
I will to honor you,
my Goddess.
I will to serve you.
I will to serve God.
Aum.

CHAPTER 16

Bring God into Visible Form through Gratitude and Faith

The gratitude series of Sacred Heart Yoga includes hatha, laya, and a deeply profound bhakti yoga. Tantra is actively alive in the heart seal, and a fusion of love exists between you and your divine essence. The kundalini surges through your heart seal, creating eternal bliss. You have entered a high state of sahaja yoga as you surrender into true union and love.

> ### TEACHING FROM JESUS
> By loving and worshipping God, you accomplish all that is needed. By blessing and thanking God, you bring God into visible form in your life. This is the path to attain all of God's wisdom and knowledge. Humankind must bring the body and soul into one force to bring the Holy Spirit through itself.

By loving and worshipping God, you feel the beauty of God and the oneness with God. What else is needed? This love and oneness is all we have ever wanted; it is what we have searched for. In this state of being, we feel incredible oneness, and we bless all of our problems, which dissolve them. They no longer consume us with worry, doubt, and fear. Our minds become clear and open to receive divine wisdom and inspiration from the mind of God. Our bodies are light, and we feel pleasure moving through them.

I have found that I am clear enough in this state of oneness that I can see my illusions, and I realize that everything is in divine order. I can bless God for my challenges, seeing that they have been what caused me to expand into this wonder of God.

Yes, my so-called problems have been my greatest blessings because they helped me accomplish what was necessary for me to move to the next level spiritually.

When I thank God for my good, I believe in God's love for me. My heart is open to give love to God and to receive blessings from God. When my ego mind says, "Where will my good come from?" it cannot conceive of the miracle because it is outside the kingdom, trapped in its limited thinking. By thanking God for my good, I suddenly move beyond my limitation; the fear is gone, and I can trust God's will to bring into form my good. Then my ego mind stops saying, "How will it come? Where is it coming from, and when will it come?" I trust that God's plan is perfect, and I don't need to know the how, where, and when. This, for me, is freedom. Joy is in my heart, and excitement fills my soul as I wait to see the miracle come into form. It is just like waiting to open my perfectly wrapped Christmas presents. As you thank God for loving you, love multiplies in your life. If you want to increase any good in your life, thank God for the good, and it will multiply. Jesus calls this the law of multiplication.

The Path to Attain All of God's Wisdom and Knowledge

By loving, worshipping, blessing, and thanking God, we become God. This practice dissolves the ego mind, which is the lack of self-love, lack of self-worth; it is guilt, regret, remorse, pain, and fear. These limited feelings and thoughts create separation from God. As we become one, we become as God is: full of love, grace, goodness, wisdom, knowledge, and power (all that we really are). Remember, we have been told we already know everything, and we will experience knowing through loving, worshipping, blessing, and thanking God.

As you practice loving, worshipping, blessing, and thanking God, the soul is purified, and the body begins to hold a higher vibrational rate. The body begins to clear cellularly. The body and soul then become one force, which allows the Holy Spirit to move freely through the body. The ego is tamed of its needs for physical, emotional, and mental gratification. The needs and addictions of the body will dissipate because the feelings and experiences of beauty, love, and pleasure that come from bringing the Holy Spirit through you feel so much more gratifying than the needs of the body.

It takes practice to change the way you relate to the force of good in the universe. As you thank God for your good, you are accepting good to flow to you. Good is all around you. Thanking God for your good draws it to you. I invite you to become still and focused within, and then repeat this prayer of thanksgiving until you feel the quickening in your soul. Choose an area for which you are thankful, and fill in the blank.

I thank you, beloved God, for_____.

Even though you may not immediately feel the quickening within yourself, I encourage you to continue the practice, and one day you will have the experience of bringing God into visible form through thankfulness.

Faith and Thankfulness
JESUS SPEAKS

Thank God for the blessings he bestows on you. Stay in the state of thankfulness. Do not repeat your request. Stay focused in the state of thankfulness, expecting God's good to be delivered to you. This is the path to attaining wisdom and knowledge. This then leads to the law of faith.

When you thank God for your good, desire becomes implanted in your soul, and the vibration of your soul is quickened through the law of faith. God is life, and when you have faith, it allows God to dissolve your fears and bring into form your desired result. You must believe that the Father within will bring you what you have asked for. Thank him for bringing this gift to you. When you have faith, you trust God and the Father within.

As you move into your own Christ consciousness, surrendering the old ways of being, have faith that the Father within shall bring you into the kingdom of heaven — into the true joy and abundance of life.

You must have faith and know all things are possible with God. If you live the life of truth and love, knowing and believing, nothing will be denied you, and all will be possible. If you believe that you can become a Christ and have faith doing the work of the Father, you shall do greater works than I.

The secret of life is achieving at-one-ment in consciousness and holding firmly and purely to the truth. Faith, faith, faith — no doubt, no fear. Blessings to you, and walk in faith.

I invite you to develop your faith and live in the state of expectancy. Expect good to be in your life by thanking God for it, even before it arrives. Faith is what allows you to heal. Faith is what brings your dreams into form. Faith is the state of allowing. Allowing God to love you is a form of self-love. When we love ourselves, we let ourselves have what we want. Then your heart is open to receive. Faith is found in the heart chakra. Jesus says, "Each must display his or her own faith to enter the kingdom of God's wealth."

Faith Becomes Knowing through Experience

In the summer of 1997, I was asked to cancel all of my traveling events during the month of July so that I could stay home and write. I lived in Palm Desert, California, where the temperatures rise to 120 degrees Fahrenheit in the summer. A large portion of the population leaves after spending the winter months in this desert paradise.

It was the perfect time to stay in and write, as the heat of the day kept me home-bound in the comfort of air conditioning. However, I had a problem since my usual clients for healings were gone for the summer and my yoga classes were over for the season: How was I to support myself financially? I soon became very fearful, so I went to my health club to take a steam. Alone in the steam room and crying aloud, I told Jesus how scared I was. He replied that he would provide for me because I was doing the Father's work. With this news, I cried even harder in relief and thankfulness. I believed him and had faith that I would be provided for. I began thanking God over and over again for bringing me the money to live.

Soon after I returned home, the phone rang with a request for a healing from the husband of a friend. Again, I felt such gratitude that I thanked and blessed God. While still in prayer, the phone rang again. This time, a woman wanted a series of four healings. I was overjoyed and overwhelmed by the results of my prayers and God's goodness. The month continued, and I kept thanking God for bringing me the money I needed. Most of the day and into the night, I wrote in total joy. The money kept coming, and it turned out to be one of the most prosperous months of 1997 for me. I completed the yoga portion of this book, and I was so very happy and fulfilled. Through the process of thanksgiving and faith, I had released a tremendous amount of survival fear.

The experience of your prayers being answered will bring you joy. Your faith and your power will grow. As this occurs for you, your prayers will be answered more rapidly. Soon, your miracles will become larger and more magnificent as you move into the state of knowing. In the state of knowing, there is no fear or doubt. Knowing is found in the seventh sacred seal.

Gratitude and Faith Postures

You have already accepted the truth that you are always loved. Now express your gratitude to God for loving you. From a seated position, bend the right knee, crossing it over the left bent knee. Sit back between your heels. If possible, keep the right knee aligned directly over the left. Place your hands on your feet, hinge from the hips, and bring your head as close to the knees as you can (fig. 37).

Feel the beauty of your body as you speak the prayer of gratitude. Feel the energy moving in the body as it comes into perfect balance, harmony, and health.

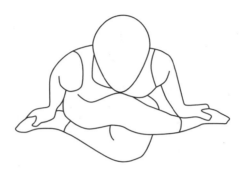

Figure 37

PRAYER
Thank you, beloved Father, for healing me.
Thank you for bringing my glands
into prefect harmony and balance.
Thank you for my perfect health.
Thank you! Thank you!
Aum.

From a seated position, bend the left knee, crossing it over the right bent knee. Sit back between your heels. If possible, keep the left knee aligned directly over the right. Place your hands on your feet, hinge from the hips, and bring your head as close to the knees as you can (fig. 38).

Feel your gratitude as you pray aloud. Feel your love and the love that is enveloping you as you speak the words. Acknowledge the love that is loving you right now.

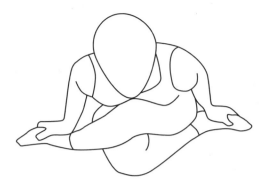

Figure 38

PRAYER
I thank you, my beloved God,
for loving me. I thank you for holding me
in the arms of love.
I thank you for filling my life with love.
Aum.

Heartfelt Gratitude

The following series of movements (figs. 39–41) is symbolic of and holds the energy of joy. The movements create within you the Essene cross as they open the pathways for the energy to flow both vertically and horizontally in the symbol of the cross. Jesus says that the Essene cross is the symbol of joy. When you are in the state of gratitude, you are in the state of joy.

The two polarities of female and male, or negative and positive energy, are joined when bringing the hands into the prayer position in front of the heart. This instantly begins to bring you inner balance.

Your knees are directly connected to the heart seal and chakra. As you kneel, the heart seal will begin to expand. You have heard the saying, "As above, so below." This is true in the body. There are hinges within the knee that open the heart. That is why, for eons, people also get on their knees when asking for forgiveness. It is because they are speaking from their heart centers. The movements that follow are intended to take you into a deep space of heart-filled gratitude, which leads you into joy.

Kneel on both knees, placing your hands together in front of the heart seal in a prayer mudra. Close your eyes, and let the heart open. Begin to thank God for your heart's desire (fig. 39).

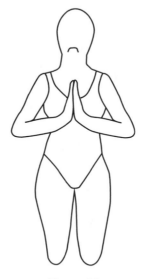

Figure 39

PRAYER
Thank you, beloved Father, for my life.
Thank you for filling my life with abundance.
Aum.

Feel the pleasure of living in the heart seal, and experience reigning in your kingdom.

When you are in the state of gratitude, you may find that the heart begins to open even more as you lean back (fig. 40).

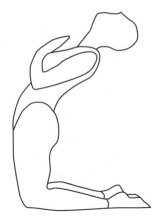

Figure 40

Once the energy has moved out through your crown seal and chakra, bow down in reverence. Bend at the hips, bringing the forehead down, and rest it on the mat as you extend your arms out in front of your head. Place your hands, palms down, on the mat (fig. 41).

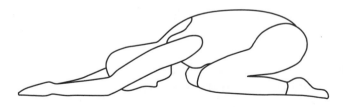

Figure 41

Begin to rest in the energy of gratitude.

CHAPTER **17**

The Principle of Being

In the being series of Sacred Heart Yoga, you will utilize hatha and laya yoga. You are living karma yoga, as the past has been resolved through your Sacred Heart Yoga practice. Your vibration has been raised above your karma, and you have been freed from your past and resurrected into love. Kundalini is actively alive within you because you have truly embraced sahaja yoga, surrender to the Divine. Tantra has woven a legacy of love throughout your entire being, and you feel whole and complete.

The principle of this series is to be available for God to love you and fill your world with the abundance of God's wealth. This state of being is you — purely you — without needs or attachments to outcomes. You are in the present moment, being loved by the God within. There is no worry or doubt. You have surrendered the fear, and you trust that God is caring for you. This is a receptive state in which you have yielded to being consumed with love.

In the state of being, there is nothing that we have to do. We have been trained in our culture to perform and compete since childhood. We are praised for how we look and how athletic, smart, and polite or well-behaved we are. The ego gets into the pattern of wanting and needing more of everything — praise, money, cars, everything in the material world — so we get caught up in needing to have success, a certain lifestyle, a certain job, and a specific kind of car. It is a consciousness in which we work to gain status through achievement: owning all the material things, having all the right friends, and belonging to all the appropriate clubs. This sets up a behavior pattern of *doing* to receive love. We begin to believe that we are loved for what we have, what we do, or how we look. We build a false perception of ourselves and of love and life. We have forgotten that our state of being is important. Even though we may have all the success and the relationships that signify that we are loved and wanted, inside there is great emptiness. We are not yet filled with God's love. Our ego still has needs to have more, whether it is love, power, money, sex, or success. We will never be satisfied until we feel we are loved.

In truth, it is not what you do that is important but how you are being while doing it. It does not matter what the task is or how mundane it may be. How are you behaving while doing the task? Are you happy, relaxed, peaceful, and fulfilled?

The truth is that you are love. You are God in individual form. You are the individual essence of your spirit.

In the state of being, you have dissolved the false concepts of self, of love, and of life. This frees you to begin to feel the God you are loving you. God's blissful energy moves up the spine into the entire body. You are consumed with your own love loving you. This love penetrates every cell in your body.

My experience of this is hard to put into words. The ecstasy of this pleasure is delicious. This energy takes me into higher and higher states of bliss, consuming me and bringing me into a state of love that is not of this world. I feel God loving me from the inside out, with every cell receiving this energy of love. In these moments of oneness, I feel safe, loved, and cared for. I need nothing from outside me. I have everything I could ever want inside of me. I can be me without the need to have anything or the need to be anything but what I am in the moment. There is nothing to prove to myself or anyone. I can trust God even more with my life, feeling that God is there loving me, filling every need I might have.

When you enter this relaxed state of fulfillment, you will begin to let the love of God dissolve areas of stress, pain, and tension that you hold in your body. You will experience this as pleasure. This pleasure of being loved is so fulfilling and overflowing that love will be expressed from you through your eyes, your smile, and your touch. Love will be in your energy field, and it will draw more love from the world around. You will exist in a river of love. God will deliver his good to you without any effort on your part. From deep within, you will have these realizations: The Father and I are one, and the Father brings me all things.

Being Postures

Sit straight and tall, extending the right leg out to the side. Bend the left knee, and bring your left foot to the inner right thigh. Keeping the back straight, begin to hinge forward from the hips (fig. 42) in blessing and thanksgiving. Let the grace of God move you forward.

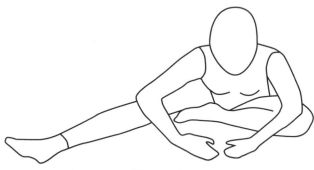

Figure 42

PRAYER

I yield to you, beloved God of my being.

I no longer need to do anything to be loved.

I no longer need to prove anything to myself or anyone else.

I am perfect as I am.

I am loved as I am.

Aum.

Let the energy move your body back to a seated position. Close your eyes, and feel the energy within and around you. Let the energy have full sway in your body as you yield to God's love for you. Again, allow the energy to move through you.

Sit straight and tall, extending the left leg out to the side. Bend the right knee and bring your right foot to the inner left thigh. Keeping the back straight, begin to hinge forward from the hips (fig. 43) in blessing and thanksgiving. Let the grace of God move you forward.

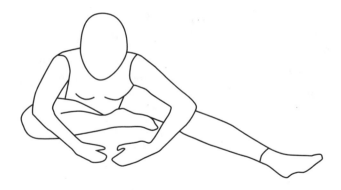

Figure 43

PRAYER
You are all that I want.
You are all that I need.
I am yours. I trust you with my life.
Consume me with your love,
beloved Mother/Father God.

Feel the pleasure of God's love for you as you allow this love to embrace you.
Again, allow the energy to move through your body.

I am being loved.
I am being held in the arms of love.
Thank you, beloved Mother/Father God.
Aum.

CHAPTER 18

Holy Communion

We come now to the final and most beautiful phase of Sacred Heart Yoga. In the Holy Communion series, you will combine all of the ancient yoga practices, and the result is immeasurable. You have became resurrected into love through the practice of Sacred Heart Yoga. Divine knowledge will flow to you as a river of consciousness to be embodied and lived.

The true, clear knowledge of gnana yoga will be experienced as you are immersed in the love of bhakti yoga, devotion to the Divine. The flow of the divine moves you into the hatha yoga postures. You have raised yourself above karma, and it ceases to exist. Your kundalini envelops you in ecstasy. Your heart gives birth to honest, deep, simple laya yoga prayers from the endless well of love you have for the Divine.

The breath breathes you as you experience pure pranayama. You will find yourself immersed in a sense of peace that is not of this world, and you will achieve a state of pure, deep meditation: true raja yoga. Yielding to the divine is easy and natural now, and you understand surrender, which is sahaja yoga. Tantra has been woven throughout the Sacred Heart Yoga experience, culminating in sweet, sweet union. You are Home at last. Hallelujah.

TEACHING FROM JESUS
Accept your divine spirit. Hold Holy Communion each day with this Divine source of wisdom and love for you. In this way, you become your divine essence.

Begin to realize that you are one with God and that the divine essence of God is within you and around you to love you always and is waiting to support you, waiting to bring you whatever you need. The truth is waiting to set you free. When we hold Holy Communion with the divine essence of God, we are given the truth to take us out of the illusion that we have been experiencing and dwelling in. As we accept the truth, we rapidly begin to move into another vibration, another reality.

We create our lives from the vibrations we transmit to the universe. We magnetize to us a like frequency to match what we transmit. As we continue to accept the truth, we raise our vibrations, and a new life is then created through the magnetized new experiences of living in love, joy, freedom, and abundance. This is all done effortlessly, for we are a new being with new truths. We live a life that is in alignment to God's will for us. We are becoming as God is: full of goodness, grace, love, wisdom, and power.

Stand in conscious communion with God, and the confusion of the world cannot touch you. The world around you may experience confusion, disaster, and even chaos. As you practice daily communion with God, you will be brought the truth of why this is occurring and knowledge of your divine purpose or the action you need to take. Clearly, you can see that everything is in divine order, moving toward peace and love. You will remain in a state of tranquility as you move through what others may view as chaos. The circumstances of life no longer own you. Therefore you can walk through the confusion in a state of certainty, joy, and even excitement, knowing something wonderful is waiting for you. As you accept and embrace the truth God brings you in Holy Communion, you will experience a new life, reborn over and over a million times.

In the state of Holy Communion, we develop the seventh sacred seal. Jesus says that within the human brain there are cells that are specifically designed to communicate with the divine mind of God. As you continue to use the prayers in Sacred Heart Yoga, you will activate these divine cells to be able to receive wisdom from the noble mind of God. We all have the ability to know all that we need to know in any given moment.

The Chakras in Holy Communion

All seven seals begin a sacred movement in this practice of Holy Communion. Jesus calls this movement "sacred matrimony," the creation of heaven and Earth within you. Each sacred seal is a pyramid-shaped symbol. In the lower three seals, the pyramid faces downward. In the upper three seals, the pyramid faces upward. In the heart center, there are two pyramids, one facing downward and one facing upward (fig. 44).

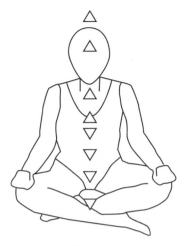

Figure 44

The purpose of Holy Communion is to create sacred matrimony, a union between heaven and Earth within you. As you move into the state of Holy Communion, the purpose is to flip the pyramids so that the lower pyramids face upward, releasing life force into the body, and the upper pyramids flip downward, bringing the divine flow into the body. Simultaneously, these two energies meet in the heart, causing the two pyramids in the heart seal to flip, forming the Star of David (fig. 45). In the moment that the energy of your divine essence and your life force join in the heart, the Star of David begins to spin, creating a combustion of energy that leaves your heart center in a spiral.

When I experienced this holy moment, it was beyond anything I had ever known. I was by myself doing my yoga in Hawaii. Suddenly, the energy began to ascend, which was usual for me. In the past, the energy went all the way up and out of the crown chakra. But on this day, the energy also began to move downward toward my heart. The two energies met, and the resulting light was a burst of power in my heart seal that spun round and round, leaving my body as a combustion of light with a force that was new to me.

As soon as this occurred, I was told that a holy matrimony had taken place within my physical body, joining my human self with my divine self and creating the union of heaven and Earth within me. A great sense of oneness and peace has been with me ever since. I am no longer separate from my divinity, and I have access to information and wisdom that was not possible before.

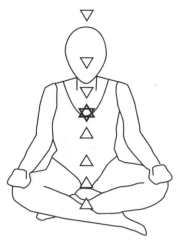

Figure 45

Conserve Your Life Force from Leaking

Every time you think that something or someone outside of you is the source of your good, your happiness, or your financial abundance, you leak your life force. Your body weakens and your emotions become unbalanced, and many times you feel emptiness or a sense of lack, loss, loneliness, or even being unloved. Every time you feel out of control or powerless because you have allowed someone else to take your power away through force, manipulation, or the fear of losing their approval, you deplete yourself of joy, power, and life force energy. You begin to feel helpless, hopeless, submissive, powerless, and even desperate. When you have those feelings, the pyramids face downward and the energy is leaving your lower chakras. You are literally bleeding away your life force.

When you look at anyone or anything — such as an attractive person or a new car — and lust after them, wanting to possess them, you again leak your life force energy. The energy leaves your body and goes directly to the person or thing. Having or desiring wonderful people or things in your life is not the error here; it is when you lust for someone or something outside of you because you don't feel you are enough that you hold an error in your consciousness. You think that you need more than you to be whole.

When you engage in these forms of third-dimensional reality, the energy from the lower chakras leaves the body and goes to the person or object through attraction. The person or object now has a part of you, and an energetic cord is established between you two. If the energetic cord is with another person, you often find yourself angry with them for controlling you or not loving you. You might even spend years trying to dissolve this energy cord.

As you evolve and heal, you enter a state of conserving your life force. You look within yourself for your good, and the lower seals and chakras feed you life force, rejuvenating your body. This is because you love yourself, respect yourself, and like who you are.

The myth that you need to be celibate to conserve life force is not necessarily true. You can enjoy a physical relationship when you realize that your partner is not the source. Under this condition, you can experience tantra with a partner, allowing the life force within the bodies to ascend through the seals and chakras and out the top of the crown.

TEACHING FROM JESUS

When you become set in lower consciousness and continue to look outside of yourself for nourishment, for love, and for pleasure, then you begin to age and die. The lower vibrations of your limited thoughts become set, and the new cells are thrown off instead of the old. The old cells then begin to decay and decompose, and you age. If you continue to receive the truth of God and embrace this truth, you will then conserve your life force, and you will live a long, healthy life because the old cells are replaced by the new cells and their vibrations of life and truth.

The key to our development is to learn to allow the life force to come up into the body to regenerate and rejuvenate us. This is obtained by accepting all of our human self — our feelings, our thoughts, and our shortcomings — without judgment. Accepting our divinity as part of us in every moment is equally important, as is accepting that we are not alone. The Mother/Father God is around us always, supporting and loving us, and is within us and is us.

Close your eyes and say this prayer until you feel the Mother/Father within and around you. In this way, you will experience the truth within.

PRAYER
The Mother/Father God is within me,
and I am within the Mother/Father God.

As we accept ourselves with our shortcomings, we no longer deny ourselves life. This opens the flow of life force energy within us, which begins to awaken the body to new life. When we deny our feelings, we are literally dying.

As we accept our humanity with all of its unconsciousness, we move into a state of wholeness. We cannot be holy until we are whole, until we are receptive and loving to ourselves exactly as we are. Remember, the Mother/Father God is here to support all of life, and we must open the gateways within us to allow ourselves to receive and manifest the wisdom of the Father and the love of the Mother in our lives.

You will find oneness, wisdom, knowledge, and clear guidance in Holy Communion. A deeply felt connection to the source will be experienced. You will experience a sense of stillness, of peace. As I lead my classes into this state, Jesus always says to me, "Peace, be still." You may hear direct communication on how to proceed with life from this source, and you may feel consumed by the grace of God. Some feel the kundalini energy rise up the spine. If you are one who has inner vision, you will see the beauty of God's life.

> ### TEACHING FROM JESUS
> Calmness, knowing, and power come from oneness with the Father God within. Oneness is the greatest power, the greatest security.

After completing the Sacred Heart Yoga and entering the final phase of Holy Communion, you will be very clear and in a state of oneness with the God within you and around you that sustains all of life. You are now available to receive the wisdom necessary in your life. You begin to have your own conversation with God, asking for clarity on any issue of concern.

You will want to stay in this state forever. Do stay awhile, for the body must be at peace to heal. You will heal very deeply in body, mind, and emotions as your spirit becomes more alive in your body. This develops your lightbody. You are becoming the light of God.

The Holy Communion Series of Postures

There are three phases in this series of postures and prayers. In the **first phase** of this posture, we bow to our humanity. Sit in a half lotus or in sukhasana position. Place your hands on your knees with your palms facing up. Touch the thumb and the middle two fingers together. This connects the flow of energy known as the kundalini. Close your eyes, and focus on the energy along both sides of the spine. Let your body sway as the energy begins to ascend up the spine. When you touch your thumb (which is neutral) to the inner two fingers (one is positive and the other is negative), you plug yourself in to the natural flow of your own female-male, or yin-yang, energy. Now sit with your back as erect as possible (fig. 46).

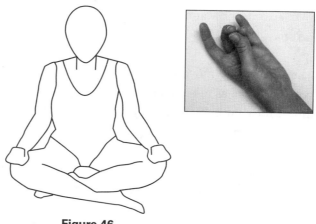

Figure 46

Hinge forward from the hips with a flat back, keeping your sit bones on the mat. Go forward as far as possible without rounding the back (fig. 47).

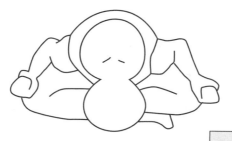

Figure 47

PRAYER
I bow to my human self.
I bow to my fearful self.
I bow to my unworthy self.
I thank you for your courage to feel your pain.
I thank you for the courage to move
through the darkness into the light.

I thank you for trusting me and the God within.
I love you, and I need you to walk
with me into the light.
I cannot go forward without you.
We are one, now and forever.
Aum.

Let the energy move your body upward into a sitting position. Feel the flow of your life force as it begins its movement up into your body. Feel reverence and gratitude for your human self as you prepare to bow.

In the **second phase** of this posture, we bow to our divinity. The posture is identical to the one used in the first phase.

Once again, sit erect. Continue to have the thumb and the middle two fingers touch (fig 46). Hinge forward from the hips with a flat back.

PRAYER
I bow to my divine essence.
I thank you for your endless
love and patience with me.
I am devoted to you, my beloved God.
I am devoted to bringing you
forth through my human form.
I give you my life.
I am yours, now and forever.
And so it is.
Aum.

Let the energy move your body, returning you to a seated position. Feel the pleasure of your own divinity loving you and blessing you as you enter the state of bliss.

The **third phase** of this posture is an active meditation. It is an acknowledgment of the female and male aspects of divinity within us as well as a time of direct communication with the divine mind of God.

Activate the Fountainhead

In the meditation for the feminine light, bring your attention and awareness down to the base of your spine on the left side. Focus on the feminine energy on the left side of the spine. You may see this as a beautiful pink light. With your thoughts, begin to bring the feminine energy up your spine, guiding it to the solar plexus and then to the heart center as you breathe into your heart. Direct the energy up to the throat and all the way out the top of your head. This creates a fountainhead for the pink light to cascade all around you. Feel the bliss of your feminine light soothing you and loving you.

PRAYER OF ACKNOWLEDGMENT
I am my feminine light.
I am the Goddess of creation.
I am the Divine Mother.
I am the Goddess.
I am the queen.
I am the priestess.
I am the purity of the maiden.
Aum.

In the meditation for the masculine light, bring your attention and awareness to the right side of the spine. You may see this as a beautiful blue light. Focus on directing the male energy up your spine to the third chakra, your solar plexus. Feel the blue light move up into the heart, filling your heart center. Direct your male energy to the throat and then all the way out the top of your head. Let the energy cascade all around you. Feel the strength and power of your male energy as it anoints you.

PRAYER OF ACKNOWLEDGMENT
I am the passion to live life fully.
I am the Father within me.
I am the will of God.
I am the king in my kingdom.
I am the priest.
I am the knight.
And so it is.
Aum.

As you complete this meditation, you have created what Jesus calls "the fountainhead." Both the pink feminine and the blue masculine light and energy come out of the crown and cascade all around the body. You are bathed in your own love and light (fig. 48).

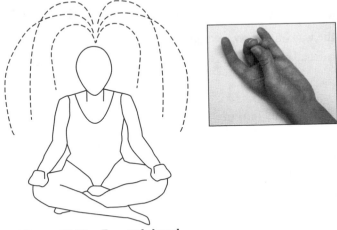

Figure 48: The Fountainhead

Enter the Kingdom of Light

Holy Communion is communion directly with God, the infinite mind. Now that the crown seal and chakra is open, we enter the kingdom of light, where all is available and waiting for us. All of the answers to every situation, problem, or challenge we may have already exist in the mind of God.

PRAYER
I enter the kingdom of light.
What do I need to see that I cannot see?
What do I need to know?

Let the answer be brought to you. Be open to receiving divine impulses of energy from God. Stay in the state of communion as long as you desire.

Thank you for joining me in this sacred moment of truth. Thank you for joining me in this blessed experience of Sacred Heart Yoga. I love you and thank you for the divine essence you bring to life.

Peace be with you. Namasté.

Experiences Along the Way

I found the way home, and I am so grateful to Jesus, the indwelling God, and Sacred Heart Yoga. Jesus has been teaching me since he first appeared to me in 1989, and I have been stretched beyond my limited mind. In early 2005, Jesus told me that one day he would manifest in my body and live from within me. Then he would manifest in physical form and teach us in small groups. He proceeded to explain that I would raise my vibration to be in union with him.

TEACHING FROM JESUS

I am the light within you. The light of the Christ is the pure principle of light that moves and expresses through an individual. You incarnated to become a living Christ and to lead your people home as I did. This is how I will come again: through those who are ready and willing to become the pure pristine light of life and God.

Well, let me tell you, I didn't believe that this was possible. It sounded like a *Star Wars* script, and I didn't buy it at all. I have always been the doubting Thomas and one of Jesus's most resistant students.

Shortly after Jesus gave me this message, I found myself sitting in a Unity Church during the holiday season. A Jewish member of the congregation was sharing the sacred traditions of the Jewish holidays. When she lit the menorah candles, I began to cry, and the voice within me said, "I am Jewish, and I have always been Jewish." This message was so strong that I knew it was true. I began attending meditations from a Jewish rabbi.

In the spring of 2006, I was again sitting at the same church, waiting for the minister to introduce me before I led a workshop after the service. Again, the voice spoke from within my third sacred seal. The voice repeated over and over throughout the hour-long service, "I am Jesus, and I have come again." The power in my body began to build, and I felt Jesus within; I felt his power and love. I knew I wasn't channeling and that this was a new experience, the one he had spoken of: the Christ light within.

I was amazed to observe and feel the Christ light taking over my body. When I walked out of the church quite stunned, a woman in a wheelchair came up to me, and we had an energy exchange. This also was a very different experience for me, for I had never before drawn physically challenged people to me for comfort and love. Then I went into the bathroom, and when I came out of the stall, to my surprise, there was a young woman standing there. She was wearing a leg brace and could not speak — results of a stroke. As the young woman looked into my eyes, I could feel the love pouring out of me, and suddenly she was in my arms crying. As I held her, I knew that the Christ light really had come again.

Later that year, I was having an *Activation of the Sacred Seals* retreat. On the last day, just before the initiation began, I was to anoint each person, assisting them to activate and give birth to the Christ within. I suddenly heard the same profound words coming from within me, but I was too embarrassed to speak them aloud. I didn't want the others to think I thought of myself as someone great, so I said the words in my mind as I anointed the first initiate. I moved to the second initiate while the energy in my body built. I spoke the words in a whisper, and as I did, the power began to fill my body. As I moved to the third initiate, I spoke the words out loud, and the Christ light manifested in my body. The Christ light remained in my body during the rest of the morning's rituals.

By noon, my back was aching, right behind my heart chakra. We broke for lunch, and I was in need of rest. A few of the beloved angels attending the retreat gave me some bodywork. I began to cry deep sobs as I returned to my mother's womb, feeling unwanted. This had been the aching in my back. I knew that the process of Christ manifesting in me was well on its way.

Another year passed, and during a level ll *Sacred Heart Yoga* retreat in my home, I awoke very early and was drawn into the retreat room. As I lay down to begin my practice, I began to speak in tongues and physically shook as my frequency kept rising higher and higher. I cried tears from deep within as I proceeded to speak and sing in tongues. I had absolutely no idea what I was saying or why I was crying, yet it came from deep within me. Suddenly, I began to remember who I was, and the yoga seemed to be complete. I walked to the altar and gave thanks. When I turned around, there were three of my Sacred Heart Yoga teachers sitting nestled on the floor in stillness. They were crying, and my body trembled as I began an ancient dance that addressed each one in reverence and love.

As the week went on, each day was more incredible than the next. I was to initiate each into the Brotherhood of Light. As the ceremony began, I went into a very high state of consciousness. I do this very often; however, this time when I opened my eyes, the veil was completely gone, and I remained in a pure state of being. (I will do my best to describe this pure and perfect state of being.) I was as light as a feather, my cells felt soft, and I moved with much ease and grace. It was effortless to exist, and I felt as if I were perpetual beauty and grace. As I gazed at each blessed one, love emanated from every cell of my body. One by one they each came into my open arms. Tears fell down my cheeks as I loved each one from a deep, pure, rich, and all-encompassing love. I was in heaven on Earth. When the initiation was complete, I knew I had found my way Home. Tears of joy released from a deep place within. We all experienced living in the fifth and six dimensions.

Wearing the Garment of Light

"As a Christ, you will wear a garment of light," Jesus told me in 2007. This garment is your radiant body. It dwells within you and radiates a light around you. The radiant body is the Christ light that heals and brings heaven to Earth, which we call miracles or manifestation.

I began to know the beauty that I am, to see the God in me, and to feel the love and beauty of God as it expresses through me. It is the most magnificent thing I have ever felt. Words cannot describe the beauty and love that flows through me to others.

I am finally beginning to know who I am and — most importantly — my worth. I am the light of God's perfect love and perfect wisdom. This light that dwells within me seems to know exactly what to do and say in the face of anger, sickness, or other upsets. It knows how to heal others no matter the circumstance. This beautiful being that dwells within me is giving me all things that I need to continue to fulfill my purpose.

It is my greatest joy to share Jesus's teachings with you. May they inspire you, enlighten you, and heal you as they have me. Following are some of the many experiences that have occurred since then. I moved to Arizona in the spring of 2010 and was guided to attend a Unity Church. I went to my first Sunday service and was welcomed with a loving embrace by the community. After the service, I was invited to join five other woman for lunch. We had a wonderful time and shared ourselves for well over two hours that afternoon.

On Wednesday around 4PM, my phone rang with an invite to a play. Because one of the women was unable to go, I was given the ticket as a gift. I was in the middle of unpacking and asked the God within whether it would serve me to attend, and I got a very strong yes. Quickly I got cleaned up and was at the playhouse by 6PM. I found my community of new friends and joined them at a table where we shared a few snacks before the performance.

The woman I sat next to told me the story of how she had fallen in her driveway right before coming to the playhouse. After she fell, her friend who was with her was unable to stop the bleeding for quite some time and wanted to take her to the emergency room. Her spirit is strong, so she told her friend that she would go after the play. She was determined to have a good time with her friends and enjoy the performance.

She wore a bandage over her right eye, which was on the side I was sitting on. I asked her whether she would like me to give her forehead some energy. After she replied, "Yes, please," I placed my right hand over the wound on her forehead and my left hand on her back behind her heart center. Immediately after I laid my hands on her, I felt a great surge of energy well up inside my heart, and I saw in my third eye the energy cross over the wound to create stitches. This whole healing energy experience did not take more than a few minutes. I removed my hands, and she said that her whole body was filled with light and that she felt fabulous.

Then she told me that she had also injured her right hip during the fall and was unable to walk without holding on to her partner's arm, so she asked me to also work in this area. I placed my hands on her right hip, and this time not only was there a surge of energy that welled up from deep within me but also a voice — the voice of the Christ-self. I heard it speak from within my heart. It said, "I fill you with my peace." The energy of peace healed her hip, and she was able to walk without assistance or pain. She was so excited about her miraculous healing experience that she began to tell her friends.

A friend who heard her story at a Course in Miracles group called and made an appointment. He arrived at my home with his wife, and they asked lots of questions. This particular man was scheduled for bladder surgery in a few days. He had cancerous cells in his bladder and wanted a healing. I told him that I had no control over the energy and that I could not guarantee the results. He agreed to give it a try and got on the healing table. I began the session, and when I got to his bladder, I saw that it was gray; then suddenly the energy began to leave my body, and I saw his bladder turn pink.

Again I heard the voice of the Christ speak, and it said, "They will find nothing abnormal." I reported to him what I had heard, and he left. A few days later, I got a phone call from him. He was elated and told me that they had found nothing. These two experiences were proof to me that indeed the body of light and miracles were growing strong in me and living through me.

My Mission in Truth

I finally realize that the path with Jesus and sharing what he calls "a mission in truth" is my life, and I want no other life. My personality self is dissolving along with my attachments to the material world. This path gives me everlasting life, what is real and true. I am filled with passion and joy, and I live in the light of the heavenly realms as I share it with others.

It is my greatest joy to serve the holy of holies. I have no life separate from this holy place within me. It is my life, and it lives and expresses through me as I continue to resurrect my ego.

About the Author

Virginia Ellen is a modern-day mystic and a bearer of Jesus's original message. She had a near-death experience in which she came face-to-face with her teacher, Jesus. In this transformative experience, Virginia was infused with the wisdom and energy to activate the sacred seals (the light in humanity). She now transmits this sacred energy to others, bringing God to life in every cell of the body while activating their sacred seals.

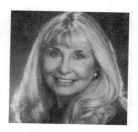

Virginia's presence creates a living opportunity to move out of one's limitations. Through her wisdom, love, and passion, she has inspired thousands to find their true selves.

Virginia speaks the Living Word of God, which transmits a sacred code of love to the listener. The energy of her words will echo in your body, creating the spin of ascension. This transmission from Virginia will cause your cells to vibrate at an accelerated speed. The spiral moves in an upward motion, and you will begin to ascend, moving back to your original light. This is the path Home that you have longed for.

Virginia is an author, medical intuitive, mystic, and coach. She founded Sacred Heart Yoga and developed the Medicine of Love: Reprogramming the Unconscious Mind method. She is also the author of *Perfect Peace: Jesus's Way to Attain Peace.* For more information, go to ReprogrammingtheUnconsiousMind.com.

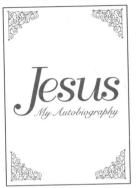
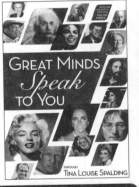

THROUGH ROBERT SHAPIRO

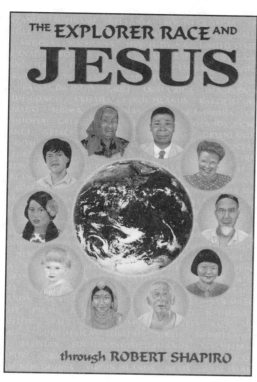

$16.95 • Softcover • 6 x 9 • 352 PP.
ISBN 978-1-891824-14-2

THE EXPLORER RACE AND JESUS

The immortal personality who lived the life we know as Jesus, along with his students and friends, describes with clarity and love his life and teaching on Earth 2,000 years ago.

These beings lovingly offer their experiences of the events that happened then and of Jesus's time-traveling adventures, especially to other planets and to the nineteenth and twentieth centuries, which he called the time of the machines — the time of troubles.

It is so heartwarming and interesting that you won't want to put it down.

Chapters Include the Following:

- Jesus's Core Being, His People and the Interest of Four of Them
- Jesus's Home World, Their Love Creations and the Four Who Visited Earth
- The "Facts" of Jesus's Life Here, His Future Return

- The Teachings and Travels
- Jesus' Life on Earth
- A Student's Time with Jesus and His Tales of Jesus's Time Travels
- The Shamanic Use of the Senses
- Many Journeys, Many Disguises

- The Child Student Who Became a Traveling Singer-Healer
- Learning to Invite Matter to Transform Itself
- Inviting Water, Signing Colors
- Learning to Teach Usable Skills

- Learning about Different Cultures and People
- The Role of Mary Magdalene, a Romany
- Jesus's Autonomous Parts, His Bloodline, and His Plans

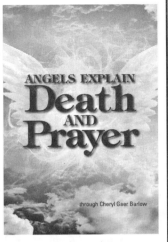
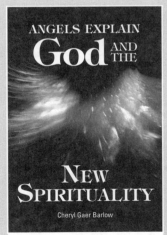

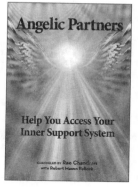
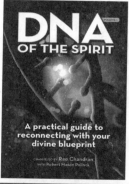
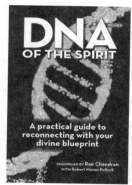

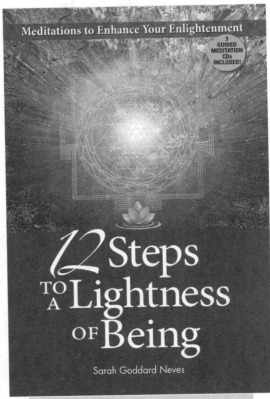
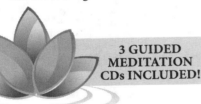

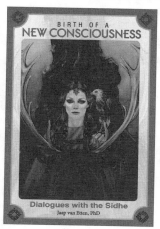
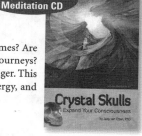
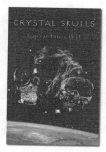
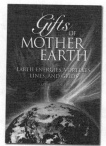

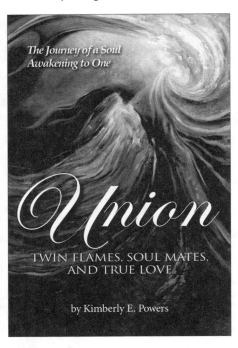
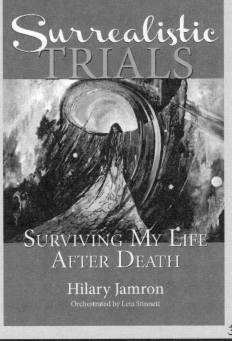

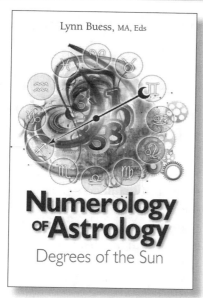
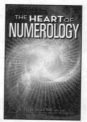
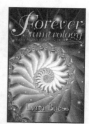
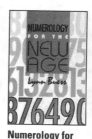
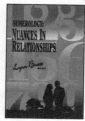
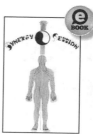
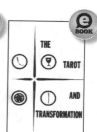

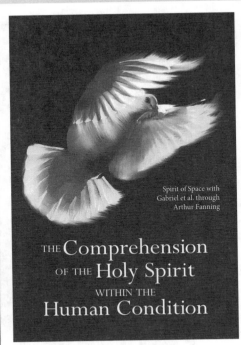
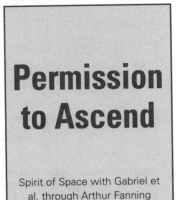
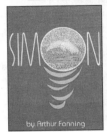
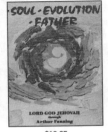

Shamanic Secrets Mastery Series

Speaks of Many Truths, Zoosh, and Reveals the Mysteries through Robert Shapiro

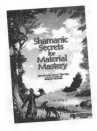

This book explores the heart and soul connection between humans and Earth. Through that intimacy, miracles of healing and expanded awareness can flourish. To heal the planet and be healed as well, you can lovingly extend your energy self out to the mountains and rivers and intimately bond with Earth. Gestures and vision can activate your heart to return you to a healthy, caring relationship with the land you live on. The character of some of Earth's most powerful features is explored and understood with exercises given to connect you with those places. As you project your love and healing energy there, you help Earth to heal from human destruction of the planet and its atmosphere. Dozens of photographs, maps, and drawings assist the process in twenty-five chapters, which cover Earth's more critical locations.

ISBN 978-1-891824-12-8 • SOFTCOVER, 528 PP. • $19.95

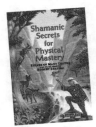

Learn to understand the sacred nature of your physical body and some of the magnificent gifts it offers you. When you work with your physical body in these new ways, you will discover not only its sacredness but its compatibility with Mother Earth, the animals, the plants, and even the nearby planets, all of which you now recognize as being sacred in nature. It is important to feel the value of oneself physically before you can have any lasting physical impact on the world. If a physical energy does not feel good about itself, it will usually be resolved; other physical or spiritual energies will dissolve it because they are unnatural. The better you feel about your physical self when you do the work in the first book, this one, and the one that follows, the greater and more lasting the benevolent effect will be on your life, on the lives of those around you, and ultimately on your planet and universe.

ISBN 978-1-891824-29-6 • SOFTCOVER, 592 PP. • $25.00

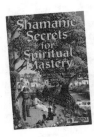

Spiritual mastery encompasses many different means to assimilate and be assimilated by the wisdom, feelings, flow, warmth, function, and application of all beings in your world who you will actually contact in some way. A lot of spiritual mastery has been covered in different bits and pieces throughout all the books we've done. My approach to spiritual mastery, though, is as grounded as possible in things that people on Earth can use — but it doesn't include the broad spectrum of spiritual mastery, like levitation and invisibility. My life basically represents your needs, and in a story-like fashion it gets out the secrets that have been held back."

— Speaks of Many Truths

ISBN 978-1-891824-58-6 • SOFTCOVER, 528 PP. • $29.95

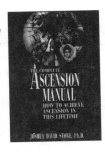
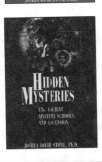
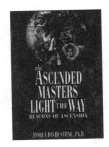
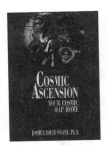
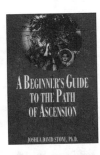
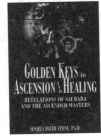

Dr. Joshua David Stone's
Easy-to-Read Encyclopedia of the Spiritual Path

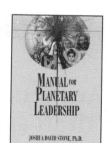
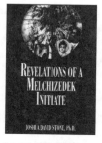
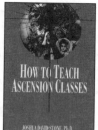
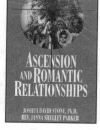
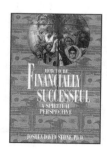
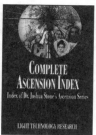
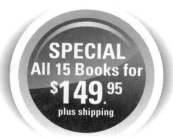

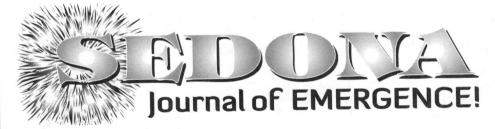
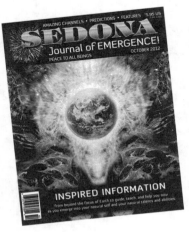